Equine Ophthalmology

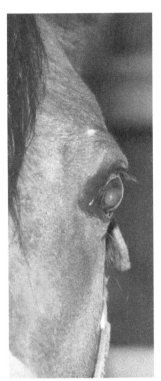

for the
Equine Practitioner
Second Edition

Dennis E. Brooks, DVM, PhD

Diplomate, American College
of Veterinary Ophthalmologists
Professor of Ophthalmology
University of Florida
Gainesville, FL.

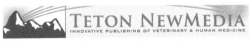

TETON NEWMEDIA
INNOVATIVE PUBLISHING OF VETERINARY & HUMAN MEDICINE

Jackson, Wyoming 83001

Executive Editor: Carroll C. Cann
Production: www.fiftysixforty.com

Teton NewMedia
P.O. Box 4833
1-888-770-3165
www.tetonnm.com

ISBN # 1-591610-400

Library of Congress Cataloging-in-Publication Data on file.

Dedication

Dedicated to the very special Dr. Bo Reich. Dedicated to all my ophthalmology residents and graduate students. I learned so much from all of you. You are amazing people and I am forever in your debt.

Dedicated to the horses: I wish I had been faster to learn.

Dedicated to Dr. Edward Mockford, Dr. Julian and Fern Krakowski, Ms Madeline Stewart, Ms Florine Laws, Ms Mae Erhardt, Omer and Doris Walton, Dick and Eleanor Seger, Mrs. Wilma Finley, Mr Robert E. Price, and Ms Marietta Baumgartner for putting up with me talking in class, educating me and having faith in me from first grade and higher.

Also dedicated to Ernie, Mel, Cola, Blink, Angie, Munchie, Travis, Spock, Katie, Smokey, Acey, Angus, Christy, Sarge, Misty, Captain, Kit, Ben, Marc, Jeanette, Gary, and Valiant.

Dedicated most of all to my Mother and Father, Betty Jane Brooks and Henry Eugene Brooks. They instilled in me the life-long desire to achieve and learn, and gave me the freedom to excel. They are the best parents a boy could have.

I love you all.

Dennis E. Brooks, 2008

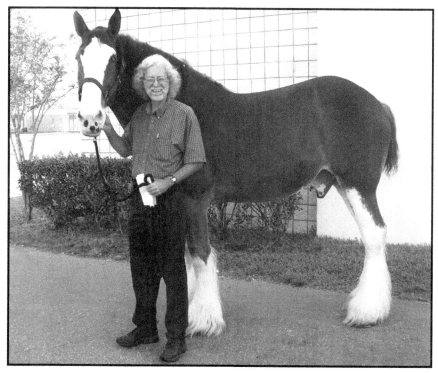

The author with a favorite patient.

Acknowledgments

Sarcoid therapy recommendations are based on discussions with the incredibly talented Dr Derek Knottenbelt of the University of Liverpool, UK. Corneal disease therapy recommendations are based on many extemporaneous and often volatile discussions with Drs Stacy Andrew, Kirk Gelatt, Dan Wolf, Tom Kern, Patty Smith, Claire Latimer, Caryn Plummer, Dave Whitley, Raine Karpinski, Mark Nasisse, David Wilkie, John Sapienza, Ken Abrams, Todd Strubbe, Kathy Barrie, Heidi Denis, Tim Cutler, Andras Komaromy, Maria Kallberg, Franck Ollivier, Diane Hendrix, Mary Utter, Noelle McNabb, Andy Matthews (long live independent Scotland!), Sheila Crispin, John Parker, Tom Miller, Greg Schultz, Mike Davidson, Dan Biros, Margie Neaderland, Dan Lavach, Brian Gilger, Yahiro Ueda, Shinya Wada, the late and missed Tadao Kotani, Carol Clark, Mike Goldstein, Jim Reidy, Phil Pickett, Cameron Whittaker, Nicole Scotty, Catherine Nunnery, Amy Baker, Sarah Blackwood, Gil Ben-Shlomo, Gysbert von Setten, and Mark Terry.

Acupuncture recommendations are based on discussions with Dr Huisheng Xie of the University of Florida, and Dr Bruce Ferguson of the University of Perth, Perth Australia.

This book would not have been possible without the assistance and encouragement of Carroll Cann and the people of Teton NewMedia.

Table of Contents

Section 3 The Equine Orbit

Section 4 The Eyelids, Conjunctiva and Lacrimal System

Section 5 Corneal Ulceration

Section 6 Other Corneal Problems

Section 7 Cataracts, Glaucoma and Uveal Problems in the Horse

Section 8 Retinopathies and Ocular Manifestations of Systemic Diseases in the Horse

Section 1

General Anatomy, Physiology and Examination of the Horse Eye

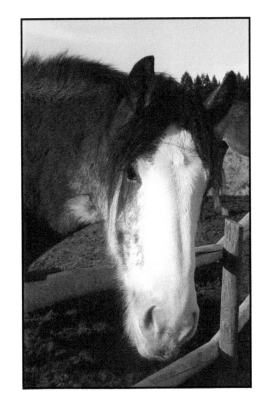

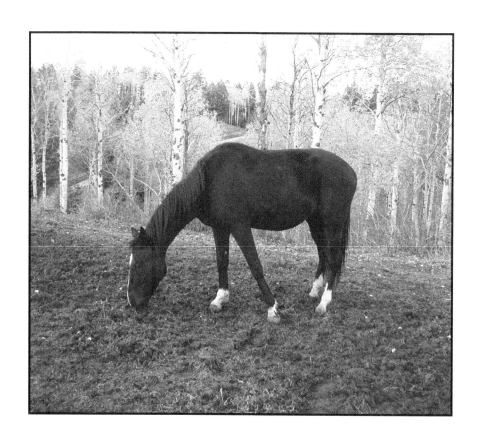

Introduction

The primary goal of this book is to help veterinarians treat simple and complex eye problems in horses. Horses are a vision oriented species in which good visual capabilities and the ability to run aid avoidance of predators. The horse eye becomes inflamed easily and often needs considerable help to speed healing. A second goal of this book is to provide veterinary ophthalmologists and veterinary ophthalmology residents a quick resource guide for the many complex eye problems of the horse.

Some Helpful Hints

The following icons are used in this book to indicate important concepts:

✓ Routine. This feature is routine, something you should know.

♥ Important. This concept strikes at the heart of the matter.

⚷ Key. This concept is a key one and is necessary for full understanding.

💣 Stop. Something dangerous will happen if you don't remember this.

✋ Stop. This doesn't look important but it can really make a difference when trying to sort out unusual situations.

⊙ The CD symbol indicates that videos related to this topic are available on the companion CD-Rom.

Anatomy

Orbit

✓ Orbit refers to the bony socket of the skull that contains the eye or globe, and surrounding soft tissue structures (Figure 1-1). The equine orbit is a large conical cavity that is closed posteriorly and has a broad opening anteriorly. The anterior rim of the bony orbit is complete in the horse (Figure 1-2). The orbit in horses is surrounded nasally by sinuses (Figure 1-3).

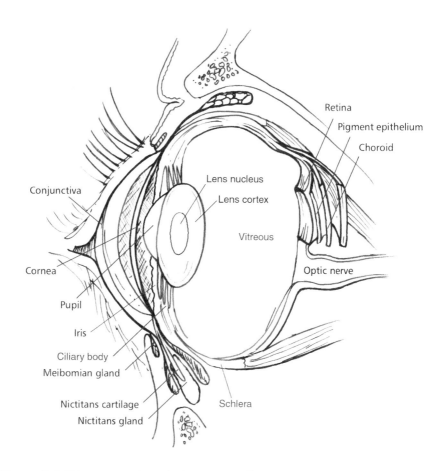

Figure 1-1 This cross-section of a horse's eye illustrates the complex anatomical relationships of the intraocular components of the horse's visual system.

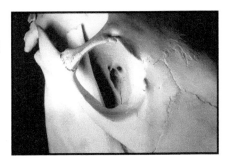

Figure 1-2 The bony orbit is complete anteriorly in the horses. The supraorbital foramen is found dorsally, foramina for passage of the optic nerve and other orbital nerves and orbital blood vessels are posterior, and the ventral orbital floor provides a soft tissue barrier between the orbit and oral cavity.

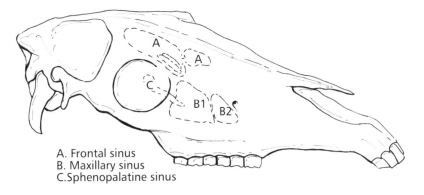

A. Frontal sinus
B. Maxillary sinus
C. Sphenopalatine sinus

Figure 1-3 Sinuses surround the globe and orbit cranially and medially. The ventral orbit is bordered by the oral cavity.

✔ The location of the bony orbits within the skull determines the degree of binocular vision. Animals with laterally positioned orbits, such as horses, have reduced ability for binocular vision and depth perception than do animals with eyes aimed more anteriorly, such as cats or dogs. Horses do, however, have better peripheral vision (Figure 1-4).

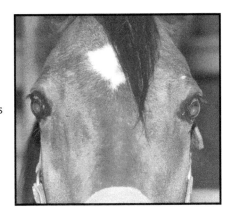

Figure 1-4 The upper eyelashes are nearly perpendicular to the cornea of most horses. Note the nuclear sclerosis of both lenses in this older mare. Ptosis or droopiness of the lid may be associated with ocular pain in the early stages of several horse eye problems.

✓ Abnormalities of the globe alone are referred to as "ocular" rather than "orbital". The area of the orbit behind the globe is called "retrobulbar". "Periorbital" indicates the area around the orbit including the eyelids, soft tissues, and bony skull.

Eyelids

✓ Anatomically, the eyelids are divided into the outermost skin, the underlying orbicularis oculi muscle (innervated by the facial nerve), the fibrous tarsal plate or tarsus, and the inner palpebral conjunctival layer (Figure 1-5).

✓ Horses have large eyelashes or cilia on their upper eyelid margin and none on the lower lid (see Figure 1-4). Meibomian (tarsal) glands, which secrete the lipid component of the tear film, are found at the eyelid margins.

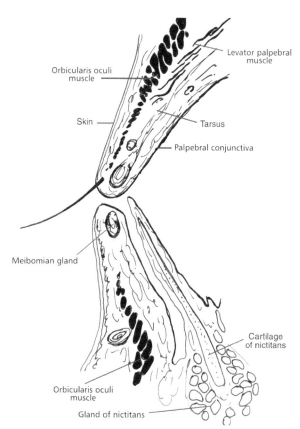

Figure 1-5 Histologic diagram of the eyelids and nictitans.

✓ Long hairs or vibrissae provide sensation in the periorbital area of the eyes of horses.

✓ The upper eyelid joins the lower eyelid at the medial and lateral canthi (singular is canthus) (Figures 1-6 and 1-7).

🖐 The eyelids are thin and highly vascular. Most (75%) of the eyelid movement is in the upper eyelid.

☞ Eyelids have several important functions. They protect the eye, produce and distribute the precorneal tear film, prevent corneal drying, pump tears into the lacrimal puncta, and help control the amount of light entering the eye.

☞ Neutrophils escape into the tear film from congested eyelid blood vessels in response to corneal cytokines produced during inflammatory corneal diseases. Eyelid swelling may thus be an early sign of corneal ulceration.

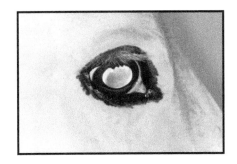

Figure 1-6 Pigment surrounds the eyelid margins in this white horse.

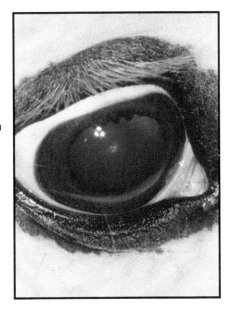

Figure 1-7 A closer view of the horse in Figure 1-6 demonstrates the pigmented lid margin, a nonpigmented margin of the nictitans, and a brown iris with prominent corpora nigra.

Nictitans

✔ The nictitans or third eyelid (TE) of the horse is located at the medial canthus. It displays rapid, near horizontal movement as it protects the cornea and distributes the tear film. The TE conjunctiva may be completely pigmented or may contain no melanin. A large gland produces part of the tear film and is found at the base of a T-shaped piece of supportive TE cartilage. Orbital fat aids TE movement in young horses (see Figures 1-1 and 1-5).

Conjunctiva

✔ The conjunctival epithelium covering the globe (bulbar conjunctiva) begins at the corneoscleral junction or limbus, lies superficial to the sclera, and reflects forward at the fornix where it becomes palpebral conjunctival epithelium. The palpebral conjunctival epithelium lines the inner eyelids and continues to the mucocutaneous junction at the lid margin. The ventromedial portion of the palpebral conjunctiva covers the nictitating membrane. Fascia beneath the conjunctiva and superficial to the sclera is known as Tenon's capsule. Components of the ocular immune system and tear producing cells are present in the conjunctiva. Conjunctiva is pigmented near the limbus in some horses.

Anterior Segment

✔ The precorneal tear film, cornea, iridocorneal angle, iris, lens and ciliary body comprise the anterior segment of the eye (see Figure 1-1).

Precorneal Tear Film

✔ The precorneal tear film is a trilayered, mucin dominated gel produced by the meibomian glands (outer oily layer), the lacrimal and nictitans glands (aqueous layer), and the conjunctival goblet cells (inner mucin layer). The tear film serves as an extracellular matrix to the cornea, provides an optically smooth surface, aids nutrition to the cornea, and contains vitamin A, proteinases, proteinase normal inhibitors, growth factors, and cytokines that affect corneal health. The equine tear film pH was 8-8.6 (mean 8.33 ± 0.15) in one study, and ranged 7.1-7.9 (mean 7.5 ± 0.5 in a second). Tears enter the tear drainage system at the medial canthus, pass through the osseous nasolacrimal duct in the skull, and drain in the nose (Figures 1-8, 2-10, and 4-11).

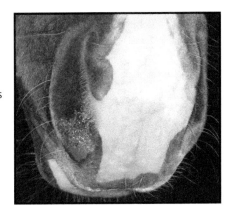

Figure 1-8 The nasal opening of the nasolacrimal duct is catheterized in this photograph, and is at the junction of the pigmented and nonpigmented mucosa in this horse.

Cornea, Limbus, Sclera

✓ The cornea is a very prominent, transparent and physically strong tissue that supplies a large part of the eye's light bending power. Light rays pass through the cornea to begin the visual process in the retina. Corneal transparency is maintained by several anatomic mechanisms: 1) the normal lack of corneal blood vessels; 2) the absence of pigment; 3) a non-keratinized anterior surface epithelium; 4) the precise organization of the stromal collagen fibrils; 5) the small size of the stromal collagen fibrils; 6) and the relatively dehydrated nature of the cornea as compared to sclera.

♥ The average thickness, based on histologic measurements, of the horse central cornea is approximately 1.0-1.5 mm with the peripheral cornea slightly thinner at 0.8 mm. Specular microscopy/pachymetric measurements yielded a mean thickness of 0.9 mm The ultrasonic pachymetric thickness was greatest dorsally, and decreased from ventral to lateral to nasal to central.

The mean horizontal corneal diameter, and mean central vertical corneal diameter are 30.2 ± 1.5 and 24.7 ± 1.5 mm respectively. The horse has four corneal layers. (Figure 1-9) The outermost stratified squamous epithelium has three cell types (superficial squamous cells, wing cells, and deeper basal cells). This layer is a barrier to the precorneal tear film. An epithelial basement membrane attaches the epithelium to the stroma. The stroma constitutes approximately 90% of the corneal thickness and is mostly collagen. Descemet's membrane is the basement membrane secreted by the inner corneal endothelium and is produced throughout life. Its thickness is only about 21 μm or the summed diameter of three red blood cells! The innermost endothelium consists of only one cell layer with the mean density of cells declining from nasal and temporal, to central, to dorsal to ventral. A higher endothelial cell density is found in

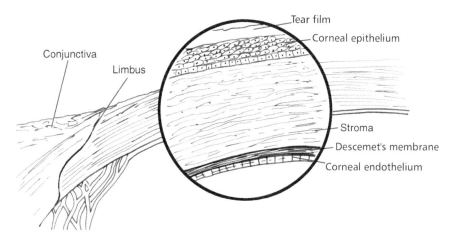

Figure 1-9 Histologic diagram of the normal horse cornea.

male horses. A sodium ATP-ase pump in the endothelium is very important in maintaining corneal transparency. Endothelial disease results in pump failure and corneal edema.

✓ The anterior cornea has a higher capacity to collect and hold water than the deeper stroma. This is due to the lower prevalence of chondroitin 4 sulfate compared to chondroitin 6 sulfate in the superficial corneal stroma.

♥ The cornea is one of the most sensitive tissues in the body. Corneal nerves are branches of the trigeminal nerve and are concentrated in the superficial cornea with no nerves present in Descemet's membrane.

✓ The limbus is located at the peripheral edge of the cornea and forms the transition zone between the cornea and sclera. The epithelium of the cornea merges with the bulbar conjunctival epithelium in this area. Stem cells present here are stimulated to form corneal epithelium during ulcerative keratitis. Inflammatory cells and blood vessels enter the cornea at the limbus.

✓ In most horses there is an obvious grey line at the medial and lateral limbus that represents the insertion of the pectinate ligaments of the iridocorneal angle into the posterior cornea.

✓ The sclera is continuous with the cornea and constitutes the major portion of the outer layer of the globe. It has a high water content and is composed of collagen. The equator is the thinnest region of the sclera in most species.

Iridocorneal Angle

☞ The junction of the cornea, iris, and ciliary body is the iridocorneal angle. Drainage of aqueous humor to the circulation begins here. It appears as a porous gray band at the nasal and temporal areas of the limbus.

✓ The **anterior chamber** (AC) is the large aqueous humor filled chamber between the cornea and iris.

Uvea

☞ Composed of the iris, ciliary body, and the choroid. (see Figure 1-1) The vascular uveal tract is involved in the production of aqueous humor, the outflow of aqueous humor, nutrition to the eye, and the immune response to numerous infectious and noninfectious disease processes. It is also responsible for accommodation of the lens. The horse eye does not tolerate much damage to its uveal tissues.

Iris

The most anterior part of the uveal tract is the iris. It is very vascular. The posterior aspect of the iris rests and moves against the anterior lens capsule. Iris sphincter muscles are prominent near the pupil margin and cause miosis. Dilator muscles in the mid-iris are thin and innervated by sympathetic nerves.

✓ The iris is separated into a pupillary zone and a peripheral base of the iris. The division between the two zones is known as the collarette.

✓ In general, the iris color of the horse is brown, varying from dark brown to golden brown to yellow. Blue or white iris color may also be seen in some horses. The pupillary zone is usually darker in color and lined by a pigmented ruff, which is an extension of the posterior pigmented epithelium. Horses have a granula iridica or corpora nigra arising from the dorsal and to a lesser extent the ventral pupillary rims (Figure 1-10).

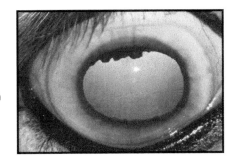

Figure 1-10 The corpora nigra and pupillary region of this heterochromic horse eye are pigmented while the peripheral iris is blue. The red reflex in the pupil is due to a lack of pigment in the retina allowing visualization of the choroidal vasculature.

Pupil

✓ The pupil changes in size with variation in environmental light intensity, being constricted in bright light and dilated in dim light. It is round in foals and horizontally oval in adults. (see Figure 1-10) The foal pupil does constrict to the adult shape when stimulated with light. The horizontal pupil of the horse necessitates that the lens possess different zones of refraction or bending power.

✓ Embryologically there is no pupil but a pupillary membrane is present. This membrane may persist in the foal and adult horse eye as a persistent pupillary membrane (PPM) (Figures 1-11 to 1-13).

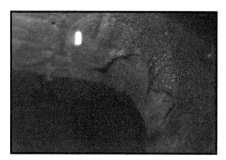

Figure 1-11 Multiple remnants of the pupillary membrane are present midway between the pupil and base of the iris.

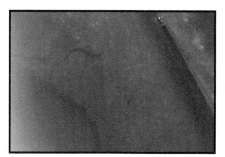

Figure 1-12 One PPM is present in this view.

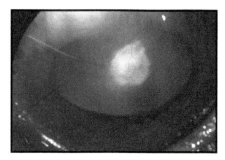

Figure 1-13 Several PPM touch the cornea to cause a permanent vascularized opacity.

Ciliary Body

✓ The middle portion of the uveal tract is the highly vascular ciliary body. It produces aqueous humor utilizing energy and the enzyme carbonic anhydrase. Aqueous humor drainage may also occur between the ciliary body and sclera (the supraciliary space) in the horse.

✓ **Ciliary muscles** are composed of smooth muscle and are poorly developed in horses. Parasympathetic nerve fibers of the oculomotor nerve and sympathetic fibers of the trigeminal nerve innervate the ciliary muscles. Ciliary muscles are responsible for lens accommodation in the horse.

♥ **During anterior uveitis** the iris sphincter muscle contracts to cause profound miosis. The ciliary body muscles undergo sustained muscular spasm to result in severe ocular pain. The interendothelial cell junctions of uveal capillaries become more permeable during episodes of anterior uveitis to cause release of plasma proteins and cells. Parasympatholytic drugs like atropine are used in uveitis 1) to dilate the pupil and reduce the chance of synechia formation, 2) to cause cycloplegia (paralyze the ciliary body muscle) which helps control pain, and 3) to stabilize the leaking iris blood vessels.

Choroid

✓ The choroid is continuous with the iris and ciliary body, and lies between the retina and the sclera. It consists of many capillaries and larger blood vessels, and is the primary blood supply to the equine retina. The triangular **tapetum** is found in the dorsal choroid of the horse. The tapetum may be poorly developed in animals with albinotic or subalbinotic coat colorations. The function of the tapetum is to act as a light amplifying device in low light conditions.

Lens

The lens is a biconvex, transparent structure located behind the iris and suspended around its circumference by zonules (see Figure 1-1). It is transparent, avascular (postnatally), and has no nerve supply. A thin, elastic capsule surrounds the lens.

✓ The volume of the lens of the horse, dog, and human is 3.0, 0.5 and 0.25 ml respectively.

✓ The multifocal lens of the horse has somewhat limited ability to assume a more spherical shape (accommodate) in viewing nearby objects.

✓ The terms nuclear, cortical, subcapsular, and capsular describe the location of a lesion in the lens from the lens center outward (the lens nucleus is the center of the lens; the anterior and posterior cortices are both external to the nucleus). The terms axial (central) and equatorial (peripheral) describe relative distance from the central axis of the lens. The anterior and posterior ends of the central axis are termed "poles".

Posterior Segment

✓ Vitreous, retina and choroid compose the posterior segment or fundus.

Vitreous Chamber

✓ The large space between the lens and retina that contains the viscous, gel-like vitreous.

Retina

☞ The retina is the most complex structure of the eye. It converts light energy into chemical energy to generate the electrical signal that is conducted to the brain. The phototransductive events that constitute the visual process are extremely intricate and begin in the retina.

☞ The retina is classically described as a 10 layered structure. (Figure 1-14) Starting from the outside (sclera) to the inside (vitreous):

1. Retinal pigmented epithelium (RPE). Not pigmented in tapetal region.

2. Photoreceptor layer of rods and cones. Rods predominate in number in the horse.

3. External limiting membrane.

4. Outer nuclear layer contains the cell bodies of the rods and cones.

5. Outer plexiform layer is the synaptic layer between axons of the photoreceptors and the dendrites of the bipolar and the horizontal cells.

6. Inner nuclear layer contains the cell bodies of the bipolar cells, horizontal cells, amacrine cells, and Müller cells.

7. Inner plexiform layer is the synaptic layer between the cells of the inner nuclear layer and the ganglion cells.

8. Ganglion cell layer is a single cell layer whose axons form the optic nerve.

9. Nerve fiber layer contains the axons of the ganglion cells.

10. Internal limiting membrane separates the retina from the vitreous.

✓ The retina is the most metabolically active tissue in the body (per unit weight), as indicated by oxygen consumption. The choroidal circulation supplies the entire peripheral retina, and the outer layers of the horse retina near the optic disc. The retinal circulation supplies the internal retinal layers near the optic disc. The Stars of Winslow are a mosaic of regularly spaced, minute dark foci in the tapetum of horses. They are end-on choroidal arterioles that penetrate the tapetum to connect choroid vessels to the choriocapillaris and provide nutrition to the retina.

✓ Basically, the rods are responsible for night (scotopic) vision, and the cones are responsible for day (photopic) and color vision.

✓ The area centralis is a high acuity region of increased cone and ganglion cell density found in the tapetum dorsal to the optic disc.

Optic Nerve

✓ Composed primarily of axons of retinal ganglion cells, the optic nerve connects the retina to the visual and nonvisual centers in the brain. The horse optic disc (also called the papilla or optic nerve head) can be seen with the ophthalmoscope in the ventral nontapetal region of the fundus.

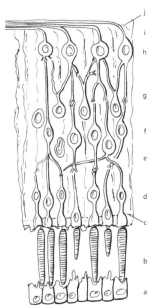

Figure 1-14 Histologic diagram of the equine retina.

a= retinal pigment epithelium
b= rod and cone outer segments
c= external limiting membrane
d= outer nuclear layer
e= outer plexiform layer
f= inner nuclear layer
g= inner plexiform layer
h= retinal ganglion cells
i= nerve fiber layer
j= inner limiting membrane

Section 2

Examination of the Eye of the Horse

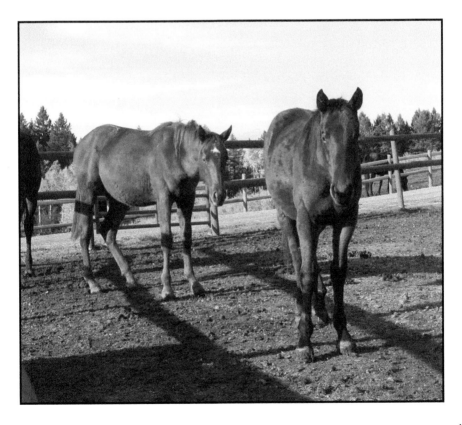

History

♥ Obtaining a thorough history is important before performing the ophthalmic examination. Painful eye conditions in horses need thorough evaluation for corneal and uveal inflammatory diseases. If some form of visual disability is suspected, it is of value to know the rate of progression of such signs, and how the horse performs under different lighting conditions. Knowledge of prior therapy is critical in most cases.

Ophthalmic Examination

✓ To be able to perform a proper ophthalmic examination it is necessary to have a bright focal light source such as a transillu-minator or a direct ophthalmoscope.

✓ The head is examined for symmetry, globe size, movement and position of the globe, ocular discharge, and blepharospasm. The general appearance of the eyes and adnexa is noted.

♥ It can be useful to examine the angle of the eyelashes on the upper lid to the cornea of the two eyes, as droopiness of the lashes of the upper lid may well indicate blepharospasm, ptosis, enophthalmos, or exophthalmos. Normally the eyelashes are almost perpendicular to the corneal surface. (Figures 2-1 and 2-2) The first sign of a painful eye often is the eyelashes pointing downwards.

Reflex Testing

♥ Making a quick, threatening motion toward the eye to cause a blink response and/or a movement of the head tests the **menace response**. This is a crude test of vision and is synomous with the term "hand motion" in humans. Care is taken not to create air currents toward the eye when performing this test. Horses have a very sensitive menace response.

⊶ ⊙ The horse should also quickly squint or **"dazzle"** when a bright light is abruptly shown close to the eye. The dazzle reflex is synonomous with the term "light perception". It correlates positively to the electroretinogram (Video 30).

✓ The **palpebral reflex** is tested by gently touching the eyelids and observing the blink response.

✓ Vision can be further assessed with maze testing with blinkers alternatively covering each eye. The maze tests should be done under dim and light conditions.

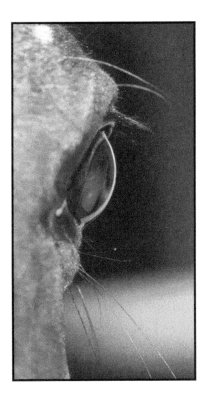

Figure 2-1 Eyelash position can aid the diagnosis of painful eye conditions in the acute stages.

Figure 2-2 Overall detailed drawing of horse face that demonstrates the lateral position of the horse globe, and the gross anatomy of the eyelids, cornea, and anterior uvea.

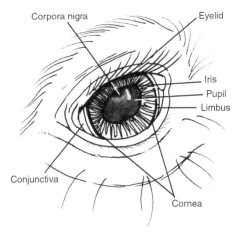

Corpora nigra

Eyelid

Iris

Pupil

Limbus

Conjunctiva

Cornea

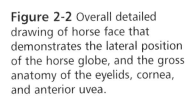 The **pupillary light reflex** (PLR; direct and indirect) evaluates the integrity of the retina, optic nerve, midbrain, oculomotor nerve, and iris sphincter muscle. The normal equine pupil responds somewhat sluggishly and incompletely unless the stimulating light is particularly bright. Stimulation of one eye results

in the constriction of both pupils. The PLR is valuable in testing potential retinal function in eyes with severe corneal opacity (Video 9).

Diagnostic Testing

♥ It is important to approach each eye problem in the horse in an ordered and systematic manner. The majority of cases can be diagnosed by using standard ophthalmic clinical examination techniques.

✓ Intravenous sedation, a nose or ear twitch, and supraorbital sensory and auriculopalpebral motor nerve blocks may be necessary to facilitate the examination.

♥ ⊙ The **auriculopalpebral nerve** (motor nerve to the orbicularis oculi muscle) can be palpated under the skin and blocked with 2-3 ml of lidocaine just lateral to the highest point of the zygomatic arch (Figure 2-3) (Video 4). It may also be blocked at the base of the ear.

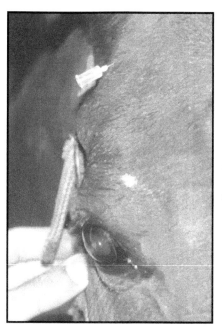

Figure 2-3 The auriculopalpebral nerve block anterior to the highest part of the zygomatic arch prevents eyelid movement required for examination or surgical procedures.

♥ ⊙ The **frontal or supraorbital nerve** (sensory to the medial two thirds of the upper lid) can be blocked at the supraorbital foramen. This foramen can be palpated medially at the superior orbital rim where the supraorbital process begins to widen. Line blocks can be used near the orbital rim to desensitize other regions (Figure 2-4) (Video 5).

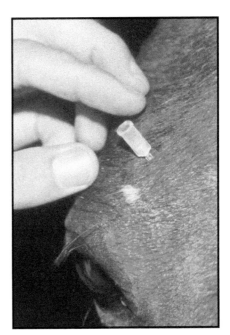

Figure 2-4 The supraorbital nerve block provides anesthesia to the medial two-thirds of the upper eyelid.

✓ **Schirmer tear testing** is a method to measure reflex tearing and should be used for chronic ulcers and eyes in which the cornea appears dry. The Schirmer tear test must be done prior to instillation of any medications into the eye. The test strip is folded at the notch and the notched end inserted over the temporal lower lid margin. (Figure 2-5) The strip is removed after one minute and the length of the moist end measured. Strips are frequently saturated in horses after one-minute with values ranging from 14-34-mm wetting/minute considered normal. Values less than 10-mm wetting/minute are diagnostic for a tear deficiency state.

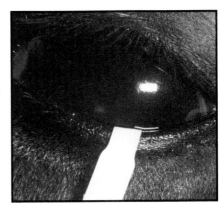

Figure 2-5 Schirmer tear test is placed in the lower lid touching the cornea to measure tear production.

♥ ⊙ **Tear Film Breakup Time:** Normal tear film is continuous. Blinking maintains the tear film continuity. The tear film breaks up if blinking does not occur often enough. Dark dry spots will appear under cobalt blue filtered light as part of normal evaporation and diffusion of tears. Fluorescein dye is placed on the cornea and not flushed off. The lid is manually blinked three times and held open to expose the tear film to evaporation. The time required for a dry spot to appear on the corneal surface after blinking is referred to as the **tear film break-up time (TFBUT)**. In a normal healthy eye, dry spots start occuring between blinks at about 10-12 seconds. A TFBUT of less than 10 seconds is abnormal and probably associated with instability of the mucin layer of the tear film (Video 15).

♥ **Corneal cultures** using microbiologic culture swabs should be obtained prior to placing any topical medications in the eye. The swabs should be gently touched to the corneal ulcer.

♥ ⊙ **Corneal scrapings to obtain cytology specimens** to detect bacteria and deep fungal hyphal elements can be obtained at the edge and base of a corneal lesion with topical anesthesia and the handle end of a sterile scalpel blade. Superficial swabbing cannot be expected to yield the organisms in a high percentage of cases (Figures 2-6 to 2-10) (Video 7). Cytology of eyelid and conjunctival masses can also be diagnostic.

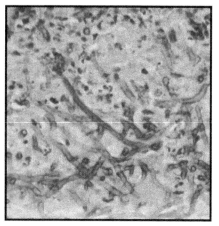 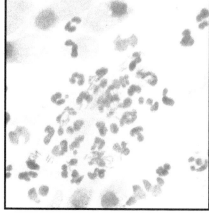

Figure 2-6 (left) Septate fungal hyphae are found in a corneal scraping from a horse with a corneal ulcer. Haematoxylin and eosin stain.

Figure 2-7 (right) Rod type bacteria and neutrophils are present in a corneal scraping from a horse with a melting ulcer. Wright's stain.

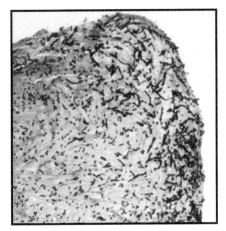 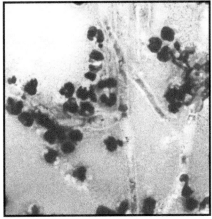

Figure 2-8 (left) Dark staining fungal hyphae are present in this corneal biopsy. GMS stain.

Figure 2-9 (right) Septate hyphae and neutrophils in a corneal scraping. HE.

Figure 2-10 Septate hyphae deep in the cornea in a corneal biopsy. GMS stain.

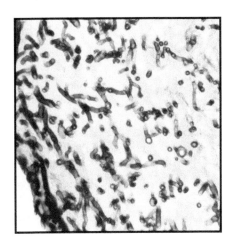

The cornea should be clear, smooth and shiny. Placing **fluorescein dye** in the eye to identify corneal ulcers should be routine in every eye examination of the horse. (Figures 2-11 and 2-12). Small corneal ulcers will stain that might otherwise be undetected. **Rose bengal dye** should be used after installation of fluorescein to evaluate the integrity of the tear film (Figure 2-13). Rose bengal dye strips are available at http://www.akorn.com.

⊙ A Seidel's test utilizes fluorescein dye to check for aqueous humor leakage through a deep ulcer, corneal laceration, or corneal suture (Video 22).

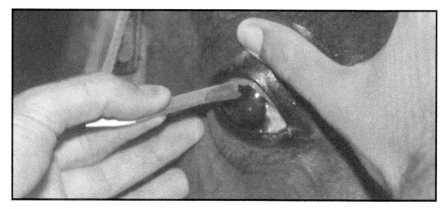

Figure 2-11 Fluorescein staining is essential for detecting corneal ulcers.

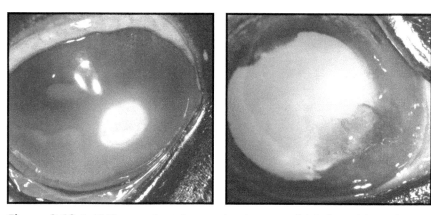

Figure 2-12 (left) Fluorescein stain retention in a superficial ulcer with moderate uveitis and early signs of stromal melting.

Figure 2-13 (right) Rose bengal stain retention in a horse with a superficial keratitis.

To determine the patency of the nasolacrimal system it is best to use irrigation from the nasal orifice with a nasolacrimal cannula or curved multipurpose syringe, although fluorescein dye penetration through the nasolacrimal system may also indicate patency (Figure 2-14), (see Figure 4-59).

The anterior chamber (AC) is best examined with a hand-held or transilluminator mounted **slitlamp** (Figure 2-15) (Videos 2, 10-12 and 23). The horse anterior chamber contains 3 ml of optically clear aqueous humor. Increased protein levels in the AC can be noted clinically as **aqueous flare** (Figure 2-16). White cells in the AC are called hypopyon, and red cells in the AC are called hyphema. Aqueous flare, hypopyon and hyphema indicate uveitis.

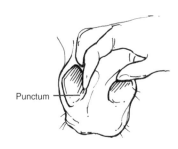

Punctum

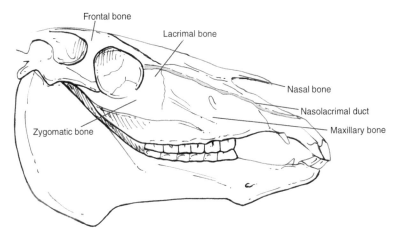

Frontal bone

Lacrimal bone

Nasal bone

Nasolacrimal duct

Maxillary bone

Zygomatic bone

Figure 2-14 Several bones form the complete anterior bony orbital of the skull of the horse. The nasolacrimal duct runs to the nasal meatus along a line just dorsal to the medial canthus and infraorbital foramen. The opening of the nasal punctum is in the nose.

⊙ The **intraocular pressure (IOP)** of horses is 16-30 mm Hg with a Tonopen applanation tonometer (Figure 2-17) (Video 8).

A **mydriatic** should be applied to the eye once the pupillary light response has been evaluated. The mydriatic agent of choice for diagnostic mydriasis is topical 1% tropicamide, which takes some 15-20 minutes to produce mydriasis in normal horses, and has an action that persists for approximately 8-12 hours. Atropine is used for therapeutic mydriasis and cycloplegia as it can dilate the normal horse pupil for greater than 2 weeks.

The lens should be checked for position and any opacities or cataract. There are a number of lens opacities which may be regarded as normal variations: prominent lens sutures, the point of attachment of the hyaloid vessel, refractive concentric rings of the multifocal lens, fine "dustlike" opacities, and sparse "vacuoles" within the lens substance.

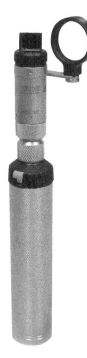

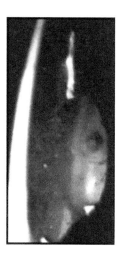

Figure 2-15 Handheld slitlamps provide useful clinical information of the cornea and uvea.

Figure 2-16 Leukocytes float in the anterior chamber in a slitlamp view of an eye with uveitis. The cornea is to the left and the lens/iris to the right.

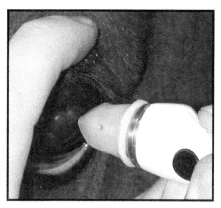

Figure 2-17 Portable tonometers allow intraocular pressure measurement in horses.

♥ Cataracts are lens opacities and are associated with varying degrees of blindness. They can be congenital, secondary to previous uveitis, and be progressive or nonprogressive. In some horse breeds they may be hereditary.

⚷ ⊙ Normal aging of the horse lens will result in cloudiness of the lens nucleus **(nuclear sclerosis)** beginning at 7 to 8 years of age, but this is not a true cataract. The suture lines and the lens capsule may also become slightly opaque as a normal feature of aging (Video 12).

✓ The adult **vitreous** should be free of obvious opacities. Vitreal floaters can develop with age or be sequelae to Equine Recurrent Uveitis (ERU). Floaters are generally benign in nature.

⊷ ⊙ The **retina and optic nerve** are examined with **direct, Panoptic®,** or **indirect ophthalmolscopes** (Figures 2-18 to 2-20) (Videos 24, 25, 31 to 35). The rotary lens setting of the direct ophthalmoscope should be set to 0 to examine the retina and optic nerve, and to a "green" number 20 to focus on the lids and cornea.

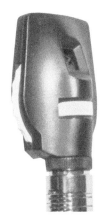
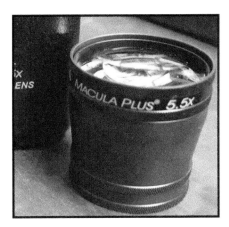

Figure 2-18 (left) A direct ophthalmoscope is required for ophthalmic examination. The lens setting of the direct ophthalmoscope should be set to 0 to examine the retina and optic nerve, and a green number 20 to focus on the lids and cornea.

Figure 2-19 (right) A 5.5 Diopter lens gives high magnification views of the horse fundus using indirect ophthalmoscopy.

Figure 2-20 The Panoptic® ophthalmoscope is an easy instrument to use to examine the horse fundus.

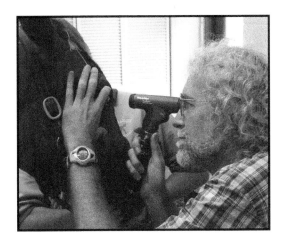

☞ Magnification of the fundic image with the direct ophthalmoscope is 7.9X laterally and 84X axially in horses, and with the indirect ophthalmoscope and a 20D lens is a minified 0.79X laterally and 0.84X axially. The image with the indirect ophthalmoscope and a 5.5D lens is magnified to 3.86X laterally and 20.1X axially; and with a 14D lens is magnified to 1.18X laterally and 1.86X axially.

✓ The Panoptic® ophthalmoscope has an intermediate level of magnification between the direct and indirect ophthalmoscopes.

✓ The fundus should be examined for any signs of ERU such as peripapillary depigmentation. The nontapetal region ventral to the optic disc should be carefully examined with a direct ophthalmoscope, as this is the area where focal retinal scars are commonly seen. Retinal detachments may be congenital, traumatic or secondary to ERU, and are serious faults due to their association with complete or partial vision loss.

✓ The electroretinogram can be useful in evaluating retinal function in horses and can be performed at referral centers (Figure 2-21).

✓ B-scan ultrasound, computerized tomography (CT), and magnetic resonance (MR) imaging are important for evaluating intraocular and orbital lesions in the horse (Figures 2-22 to 2-39).

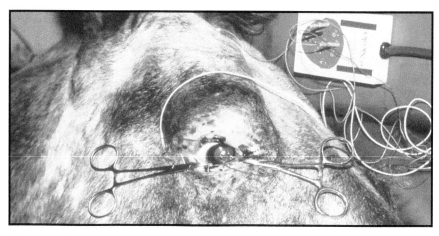

Figure 2-21 A corneal contact lens positive electrode, the negative electrode at the lateral canthus, and the ground electrode placed 1 cm from the crown of the head, are used to obtain the electroretinogram in horses.

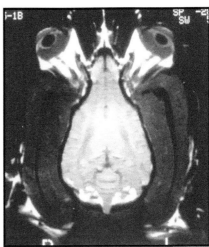

Figure 2-22 The iris, lens, optic nerve, and extraocular muscles are found in this detailed MR image of a normal foal.

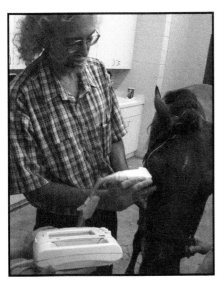

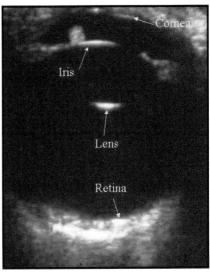

Figure 2-23 (left) Ocular ultrasound is easily performed in the horse.

Figure 2-24 (right) This ultrasound image of a normal horse has the cornea at the top and then the anterior chamber and iris; the lens is next and clear except for the bright posterior capsule; the vitreous is dark; and the retina/optic nerve are white and at the bottom. A cystic corpora nigra is present at the left part of the iris.

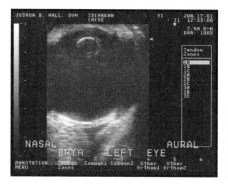
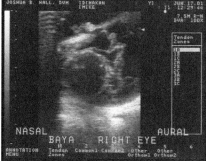

Figure 2-25 (left) The b-scan ultrasound image in this normal foal eye does not have lens, vitreal, or retinal changes. The muscles surrounding the optic nerve are prominent.

Figure 2-26 (right) A posterior lens luxation (circular structure) is found with a retinal detachment (convoluted linear opacity) in this b-scan ultrasonic image.

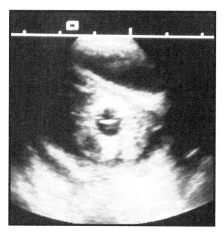
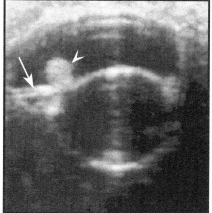

Figure 2-27 (left) The cataractous lens has luxated and is sitting in the vitreal chamber in this horse eye.

Figure 2-28 (right) The granula iridica (arrowhead) is present in this scan. The arrow marks a portion of the iris with ciliary body posterior to it.

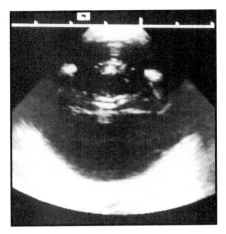
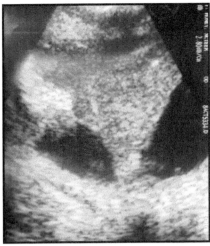

Figure 2-29 (left) Ultrasound of the eye of an old horse has some age-related lens opacification but the rest of the globe is normal.

Figure 2-30 (right) The vitreous is filled with opaque debris and the subretinal space dark due to a traction retinal detachment in this horse following rupture of a corneal ulcer. The retina is still attached at the optic nerve head.

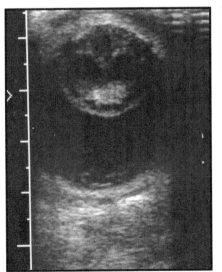
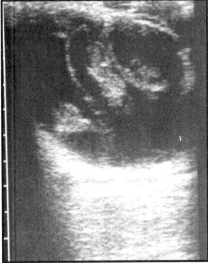

Figure 2-31 (left) Ultrasound evidence of a cataract is in this horse eye. Some vitreal debris is found near the retina at the bottom of the scan.

Figure 2-32 (right) Aiming the ultrasound probe at a different angle finds disruption of the posterior lens capsule and more vitreal debris in the eye in Figure 2-31.

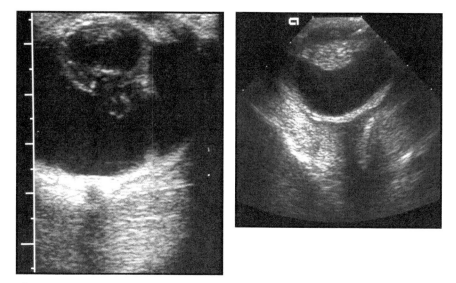

Figure 2-33 (left) The posterior lens capsule is abnormal and found to be ruptured in the eye in Figure 2-31.

Figure 2-34 (right) Ultrasound evidence of a cataract in this horse eye. This scan shows the optic nerve (dark) surrounded by the extraocular muscles (white).

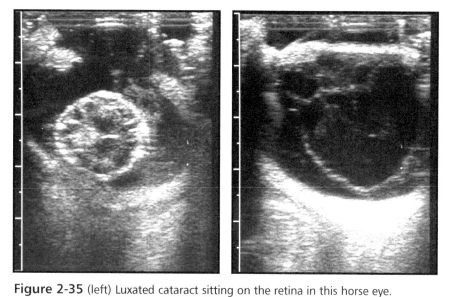

Figure 2-35 (left) Luxated cataract sitting on the retina in this horse eye.

Figure 2-36 (right) Retinal detachment is seen as a thick linear opacity near the optic nerve at the bottom of the scan in the eye in Figure 2-35.

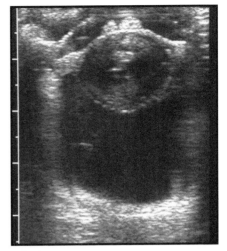

Figure 2-37 Cataract is present in this ultrasound scan of a horse eye.

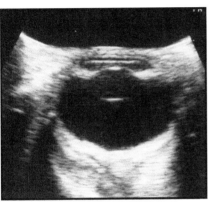

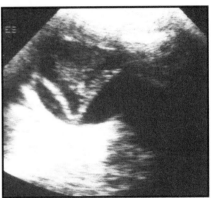

Figure 2-38 (left) Fibrin is noted in the anterior chamber of this horse with uveitis. The lens and vitreous are normal.

Figure 2-39 (right) A retinal detachment is diagnosed with ultrasound in this eye. The classic "seagull" sign is found in the vitreous.

What does the Horse "See"? Visual Capabilities of the Horse

✓ The equine eye has developed a number of unique anatomic and physiologic features to suit its special visual needs. Adaptive influences include the horse's role as a prey species, its grazing habits, and the need for arrhythmic (diurnal and nocturnal) activity. Important adaptations to avoid predators are a large visual field, and improved detection of motion. These adaptations limit, however, the ability to detect fine visual detail.

✓ The horse has a panoramic visual field of about 350 degrees and tremendous peripheral vision due to the extreme lateral globe position, the nasal extension of the retina, and the horizontal shape of the pupil. It has narrow blind spots immediately anterior to the nose and posterior to the tail. This means that a horse can just about see its tail with its head pointed forward (Figure 2-40).

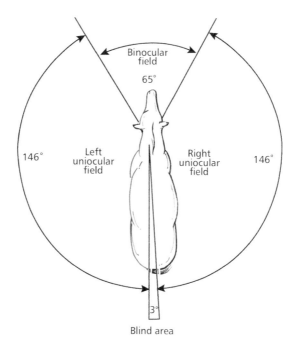

Figure 2-40 Panoramic visual fields of the horse indicate what the horse can see from one eye (uniocular) or both eyes (binocular).

✓ A small frontal binocular field of 65-70 degrees develops post-natally. The horse utilizes both eyes until an object approaches within 3-4 feet when it is forced to turn its head to continue to observe with one eye.

✓ The ability to detect differences in depth (binocular depth thresholds) is comparable to cats and indicates that horses possess stereopsis. Horses are also capable of utilizing monocular depth cues in judging distance.

✓ The horse has 0.6 times the visual acuity of humans, 1.5 times that of dogs, and 3 times that of cats. That would mean a Snellen acuity of 20/33 (i.e. a horse viewing an object at a distance of 20 feet has approximately the visual acuity of a person viewing the object at 33 feet).

☞ Horses have minimal refractive errors ranging from +3 to -3 diopters (D). Mean refractive error of horses is -1.0D. The horse has weak accommodative ability of the lens and therefore has limited near focus capability.

✔ The aphakic equine globe is +9.9D hyperopic or far-sighted. In spite of that, aphakic horses after cataract surgery seem to have relatively normal functional vision. This suggests that horses have a retinal ganglion cell receptor field size several times larger than humans do. This means that the enlarged blurred retinal image in the aphakic equine eye could still fall within the retinal ganglion cell receptor field of the horse and not cause significant loss of visual acuity.

♥ The retina of the horse contains both rod and cone photoreceptors with rods outnumbering cones 9 to 1. Rods are most sensitive to dim light and are useful for motion detection. Cones are most sensitive to bright light, are responsible for color vision, and provide good visual resolution.

☞ The area of maximal visual acuity and highest cone density in the retina of the horse is the area centralis. The equine area centralis is divided into the area centralis rotunda, a small, circular region temporal and dorsal to the optic disc, and the visual streak, a horizontal, narrow band above the optic nerve. Horses have poor acuity but good motion detection capability in the peripheral retina.

☞ Changes in head orientation, dynamic accommodation, and the presence of an area centralis aid near vision in horses. Horses need to accommodate <2D to maintain a focused image on the retina. There is thus no need for a difference in dorsal versus ventral globe length (the "ramp retina") to achieve this accommodative level.

Measurements of equine spectral sensitivity have shown a primary peak at 539 nm (greenish yellow), with a second peak at the far blue end of the color spectrum (428 nm). The horse thus sees blue, yellow and green colors, but may not see red as humans can.

☞ The fibrous tapetum of the dorsal fundus enhances night vision but probably degrades photoreceptor image resolution and thus decreases acuity in the daytime due to glare and scattering of light.

☞ The optic nerve of the horse is unique in that it contains a substantial proportion of axons of large diameter. Large retinal ganglion cells possess large diameter axons and are involved in motion detection, stereopsis, and sensitivity to dim light, suggesting that the horse has strong retinal adaptions for these visual characteristics.

✓ The equine eye also shows diurnal adaptations, such as the corpora nigra (which protects the ventral retina from excessive light exposure during grazing), occludable pupils, and yellow pigment in the lens (limits transmittance of very short wavelength, high-energy light to protect the retinal photoreceptors).

Ocular Problems in the Foal

☞ Equine neonates differ from adult horses during neurological examination in many regards. Head movements in response to auditory or tactile stimuli are jerky and exaggerated. The pupillary light response and blink-to-light response are present soon after birth. The pupillary light response may be slightly delayed in excited foals. The menace reflex (eyelid closure in response to a threatening gesture) is not consistently present in foals less than 2 weeks of age. However, by one day of age, an alert foal will withdraw its head from the menacing gesture.

☞ A newborn foal may exhibit lagophthalmos, low tear secretion, a slightly more rounded pupil that constricts to the adult shape, and reduced corneal sensitivity. The anterior and posterior Y sutures of the lens are usually visible and must not be mistaken for a cataract. The normal neonatal lens may also appear slightly cloudy for the first two days of life. Blood may be present in the hyaloid vessels for the first few hours after birth. Empty blood vessels may be seen traversing the posterior lens capsule for the first 1-4 days of life. The point of attachment of the hyaloid vessels represented by an opaque central dot just posterior to the posterior capsule may be seen for 4-8 weeks. Evaluation of sight in the neonatal foal may be difficult because the menace reflex is usually absent until about 2 weeks of age. Ocular problems occur far more commonly than most clinicians recognize. Corneal ulcers were recorded in nearly 20% of all foals admitted to our hospital. This was particularly true in certain groups of foals, especially foals with hypoxic ischemic encephalopathy and premature animals. Unlike adult animals, foals with corneal ulcers fail to demonstrate the classical clinical signs of blepharospasm, epiphora and ocular pain. The optic disc of the foal is round with smooth margins.

✔ Tapetal color is related to iris and coat color and is usually blue-green, but may be partially red, orange, or blue. Dark bay and brown horses usually have a blue-green tapetum and darkly pigmented nontapetal region. Lighter chestnuts and palominos may have a yellow tapetum with a light brown nontapetal area. Gray and white horses may have a yellow tapetal color with a light or nonpigmented nontapetal region. Color dilute foals have a red fundic reflection due to exposure of choroidal blood vessels from a lack of a tapetum and reduced retinal pigmentation.

🕭 **The Anterior Segment Dysgenesis syndrome** of ciliary body cysts, iris hypoplasia, cataracts and retinal dysplasia is found in the Rocky Mountain Horse, Connemara pony, miniature horses, and other horses with the "silver dapple" gene in the USA (see Figure 7-73).

🕭 **Dermoids** are aggregates of skin tissue aberrantly located in the conjunctiva, cornea or eyelid (Figures 2-41 and 2-42). Hairs may not always be prominent. Treatment would be a keratectomy for corneal dermoids, and blepharoplasty for eyelid lesions. Other congenital tumors noted are hemangiomas (Figures 2-43 to 2-45).

✔ **Subconjunctival and scleral hemorrhage** may occur in one or both eyes of foals delivered from maiden mares. The narrow pelvis of such mares may lead to compression of the head and globes to cause scleral vessel rupture and hemorrhage in larger weight foals. Dystocias may also have ptosis due to damage to the facial nerve during delivery. No therapy is generally indicated.

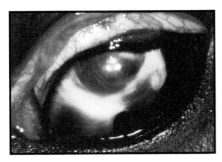 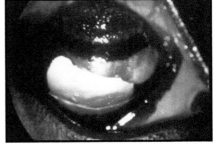

Figure 2-41 (left) A small brown dorsal limbal dermoid with corneal opacification is found in this foal.
Figure 2-42 (right) Small white glands are found in this corneal dermoid.

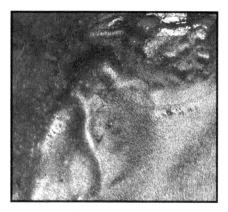
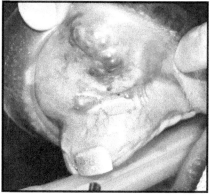

Figure 2-43 (left) Fluctuant, blood filled swellings of the lower lid, face, gums, and nasal passageways in a foal caused by a congenital hemangioma.
Figure 2-44 (right) Gum hemangiomas in the horse in Figure 2-43.

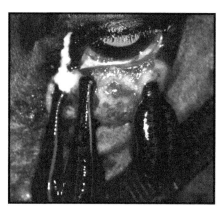

Figure 2-45 Cryosurgery, intralesional steroids, and medical grade leeches were used in the therapy of the hemangioma in the horse in Figure 2-43.

Entropion is an inward rolling of the eyelid margin. This causes the eyelid hairs to rub on the cornea. It can be a primary problem in foals, or secondary to emaciation as in "downer foals." Dehydration alone rarely causes serious entropion. It may be repaired to prevent corneal ulceration in the neonate by placing sutures at the lid margin in a vertical mattress pattern to evert the offending eyelid margin (Figures 2-46 to 2-48). Fluid injection (trimethoprim sulfa) into the entropic area can temporarily relieve entropion in some foals.

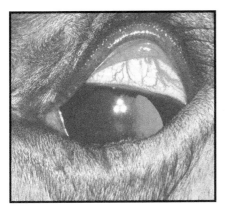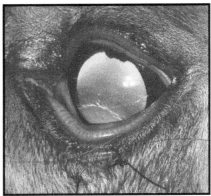

Figure 2-46 Severe lower eyelid entropion is found in this foal. The eversion of the upper lid is from handling during the photography.

Figure 2-47 Everting sutures eliminate the entropion in the foal in Figure 2-46 and allow observation of a superficial corneal ulcer caused by the entropion.

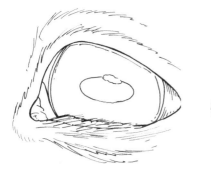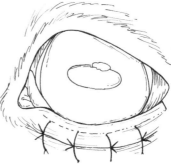

Figure 2-48 Entropion surgical repair in foals consists of placement of simple interrupted or vertical mattress sutures to roll out the affected eyelid margin to prevent hairs from irritating the cornea.

🔑 **Lacrimal puncta agenesis or duct atresia** may be unilateral or bilateral. Clinical signs are a chronic mucoid and eventually mucopurulent discharge (often copious) in a young horse. Presumptive diagnosis of duct agenesis may be made by noting a lack of a distal opening of the nasolacrimal duct or puncta at the mucocutaneous junction within the nares (Figure 2-49 to 2-53 and 4-56 to 4-58).

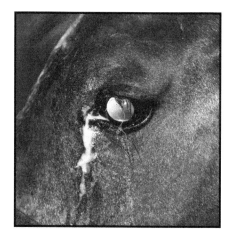

Figure 2-49 Purulent nasal discharge due to congenital nasolacrimal duct disease in this yearling.

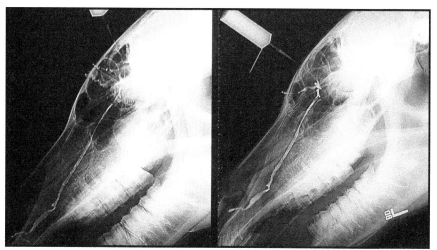

Figure 2-50 Normal dacrycystorhinograms in a foal indicate the length and complexity of the tear drainage system.

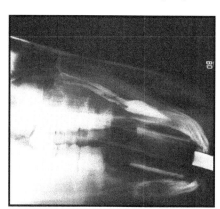

Figure 2-51 Blockage of the nasolacrimal ducts in the horse in Figure 2-49 due to absence of the opening of the duct in the nasal meatus is evident in this dacrycystorhinogram.

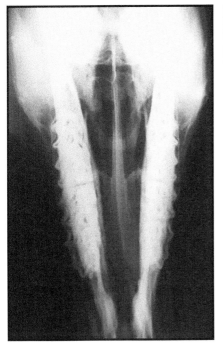
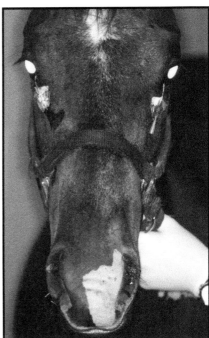

Figure 2-52 (left) Radiopaque dye stops at the distal opening of the nasolacrimal duct in the yearling in Figure 2-49.

Figure 2-53 (right) Catheter placement prevents premature closure of the surgically created nasal openings of the nasolacrimal ducts in the horse in Figure 2-49.

✓ **Persistent pupillary membranes (PPMs)** seldom cause any visual impairment although focal lens or corneal opacities may be present. There is no therapy (see Figures 1-11 to 1-13).

✓ **Congenital cataracts** in foals are common congenital eye defects. Surgery is recommended as soon as possible (Figures 2-54 and 2-55).

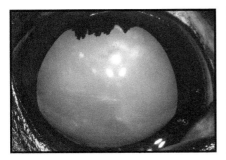
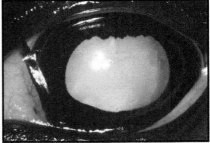

Figure 2-54 (left) Near mature cataract in a young Arabian colt.

Figure 2-55 (right) Near mature cataract in a throroughbred foal.

Microphthalmos is a common ophthalmic congenital defect in the foal. A range of lesions may be present. The microphthalmic eye may be visual or associated with other eye problems that cause blindness. The clinical appearance of microphthalmos may be difficult to differentiate from an atrophic or phthisical globe (Figures 2-56 to 2-61).

✓ **Strabismus** is deviation of the globe from its normal orientation and may be noted alone or with other congenital ocular deformities (Figure 2-62).

✓ **Congenital lens luxation** is a severe eye problem that requires surgery for resolution.

✓ **Subconjunctival hemorrhage** may be found in foals following dystocias or ocular trauma (Figures 2-63 and 2-64). No therapy is indicated in most cases as it will resolve.

♥ **Persistent superficial corneal ulcers or erosions** in the neonatal foal may be associated with decreased corneal sensation and thus be slow to heal.

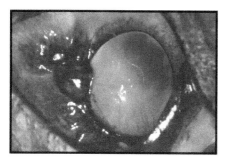 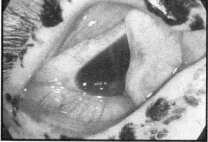

Figure 2-56 (left) A small opaque cornea is found in this microphthalmic eye.
Figure 2-57 (right) Severe trauma resulted in this atrophic, phthisical globe.

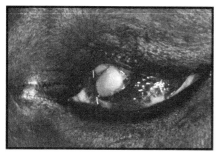

Figure 2-58 Microphthalmic globe in a foal with small cornea and conjunctival exposure.

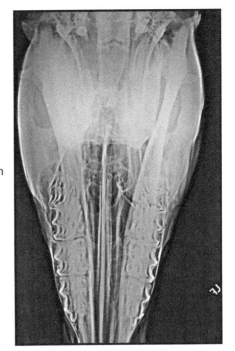

Figure 2-59 Skull deformity is associated with the microphthalmia in the foal in Figure 2-58 and noted on the right side of the radiograph.

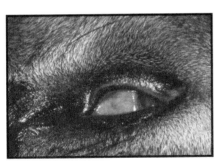
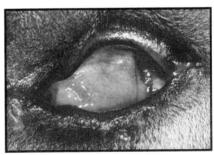

Figure 2-60 (left) Microphthalmos in this foal is associated with nictitans protrusion.
Figure 2-61 (right) Closeup view of Figure 2-60 reveals prominent nictitans.

Figure 2-62 Dorsal deviation of the globe or strabismus is present in this foal.

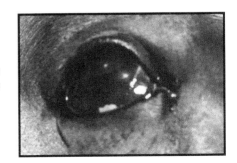

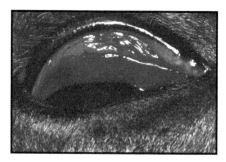 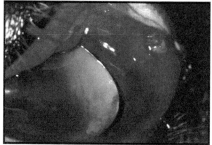

Figure 2-63 (left) Subconjunctival hemorrhage in a foal that had a difficult birth does not require therapy.

Figure 2-64 (right) Trauma to the eyelid caused subconjunctival hemorrhage in this foal.

✓ **Iridocyclitis** in the foal is generally secondary to septicemia such as Salmonella, intestinal parasites, abdominal abscesses, and *Rhodococcus*. It may be unilateral or bilateral. Fibrin, hyphema and/or hypopyon may be present. Infectious and toxic etiologies are reported in foals. Severe unilateral, blinding, fibrinous uveitis secondary to plant toxins has been noted in primarily Thoroughbred foals and yearlings in the southern USA (Figures 2-65 to 2-69).

✓ **Congenital glaucoma and congenital retinal detachment** are found periodically in foals and represent severe blinding eye problems (Figure 2-70).

✓ **Subretinal and intraretinal hemorrhages** varying from 1-20 in number may be found in up to 16% of neonatal foals. These hemorrhages are bilateral in most of these foals. Capillary rupture during parturition is a proposed mechanism for these hemorrhages which generally resolve over a few weeks with no ill effects.

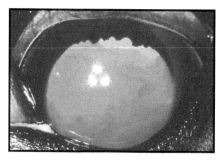 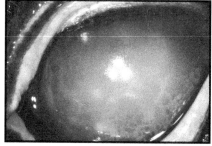

Figure 2-65 (left) Fibrin fills the anterior chamber in this foal with anterior uveitis. The pupil is dilated from mydriatic treatment.

Figure 2-66 (right) The anterior chambers of both eyes are filled with yellowish fibrin in a foal with uveitis and Rhodococcus pneumonia.

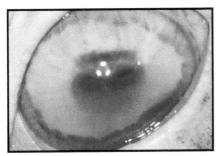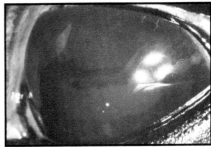

Figure 2-67 (left) Fibrin is present in the anterior chamber of a foal with uveitis. The pupil is miotic. Peripheral corneal vascularization is prominent.
Figure 2-68 (right) Fibrin obscures the miotic pupil in a foal with uveitis.

Figure 2-69 The fibrin has been digested with TPA and the pupil dilated with atropine following five days of medical therapy in the eye in Figure 2-68.

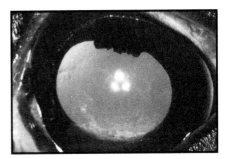

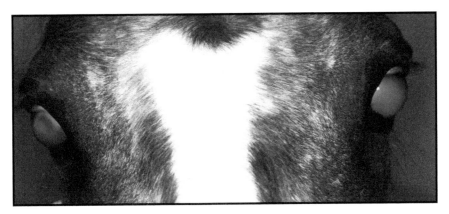

Figure 2-70 Bilateral corneal edema is present in this foal with congenital glaucoma.

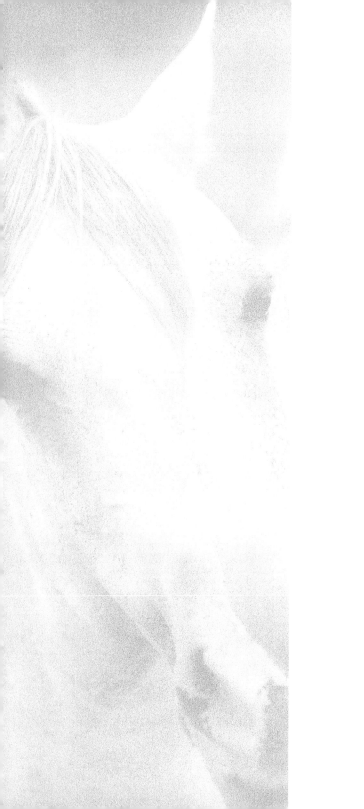

Section 3

The Equine Orbit

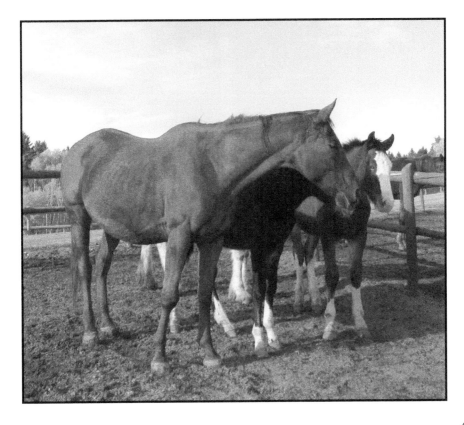

✓ The orbit is composed of several bones forming a series of canals, fissures, and foramina that contain the globe, orbital fascia, the optic nerve and other nerves, blood vessels, muscle, fat, and glands.

Orbital Diagnostic Techniques

✓ Skull radiographs, orbital ultrasound, CT or MR imaging, cytology, microbial culture and sensitivity, and biopsy are recommended as part of an orbital disease work up (see Figure 2-22, and Figures 3-1 to 3-3). Trephination into paranasal sinuses may be indicated for biopsy, microbial culture, irrigation and drainage.

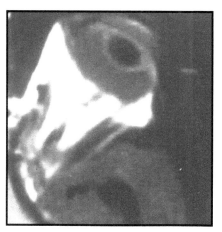
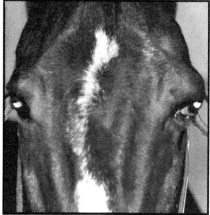

Figure 3-1 (left) MR imaging provides detailed observation of the eye and orbit. Note the iris, lens, and orbital contents.

Figure 3-2 (right) Orbital swelling neoplasia is causing slowly progressive exophthalmos of the left eye in an old Thoroughbred gelding.

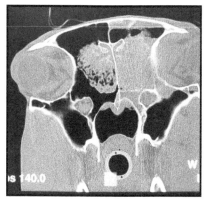

Figure 3-3 CT scan of the horse in Figure 3-2 reveals a sinus mass causing the exophthalmos.

✔ **Ultrasonography** is a noninvasive, painless procedure that can qualitatively and quantitatively evaluate various orbital abnormalities (see Figure 2-25). Diagnostic ultrasonography is indicated for evaluation of an exophthalmic globe or a globe obscured by opacities of the cornea, lens, or vitreous. This technique allows visualization of the retrobulbar soft tissue space previously only poorly visualized by other radiographic techniques. Differentiation of solid soft tissue masses versus cystic orbital masses, determination of the size of various globe or orbital components, and localization of foreign bodies is possible.

✔ **Exophthalmos**, or anterior displacement of the globe, is associated with nictitans protrusion and lagophthalmos. It can result in corneal ulceration.

✔ Exophthalmos can be confused with buphthalmos, which is a marked increase in globe diameter associated with advanced glaucoma.

☛ Infectious, traumatic, inflammatory or neoplastic disease processes involving the eyelids, the frontal, maxillary and sphenopalatine sinuses, tooth roots, the guttural pouch, nasal cavity and cranium may extend into the orbit to cause exophthalmos and/or strabismus (see Figure 3-2). Ethmoidal hematomas can cause exophthalmos. Orbital abscesses can cause exophthalmos in horses.

☛ Retrobulbar hemorrhage and cellulitis associated with orbital trauma can cause exophthalmos.

✔ **Enophthalmos**, or posterior displacement of the globe, is due to dehydration, atrophy of orbital fat, orbital fractures, and phthisis.

✔ **Strabismus** is deviation of the visual axis of one or both globes, and can be found with neurologic deficits, nystagmus, visual difficulties and abnormal head posture. In the neonatal foal, the horizontal axis of the pupil and globe is deviated slightly medially and ventrally with the eye reaching the normal adult position by one month of age (see Figure 2-62). An intracranial abscess caused by Rhodococcus is reported as a cause of unilateral strabismus and bilateral nystagmus in a young foal.

✔ Orbital asymmetry can develop secondary to orbital rim fractures, orbital cellulitis and abscesses, orbital tumors, and orbital emphysema.

✔ Congenital strabismus (hyperopia) and dorsomedial strabismus are reported in Appaloosa foals and may be associated with Equine Congenital Stationary Night Blindness. Esotropia (crossed eyes) is reported in mules. Strabismus may also result from space occupying lesions of the orbit, or be due to muscle avulsion from a traumatic proptosis.

✓ **Orbital fat prolapse** can occur from trauma or idiopathic means (Figure 3-4).

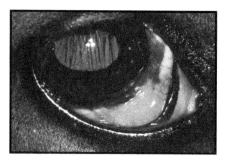

Figure 3-4 Orbital fat prolapse can resemble conjunctival tumors.

Orbital Trauma, Contusion and Periorbital Fractures

✓ Horses may injure the orbital region on the race track, in trailers or pastures, by rearing and hitting stall ceilings or starting gates, from gunshots, kicks from other horses, or when being disciplined.

✓ Periorbital fractures of the orbital rim, zygomatic arch and supra-orbital process can occur from collisions with inanimate objects, or from kicks or blows to the head. Orbital fractures, panophthalmitis, globe rupture, and orbital cellulitis and abscesses can result from orbital trauma (Figures 3-5 to 3-10).

✓ The iridocorneal angle may separate or collapse in eyes that have suffered blunt trauma to the globe. These traumatic angle changes may also be associated with retinal hemorrhages.

✓ Long term damage may be sustained in orbital trauma, including eyelid paralysis, chronic keratitis, or intermittent nasal or ocular discharge.

☞ **Orbital fractures** can be identified by palpation, facial deformity, and radiography. Blepharedema, epistaxis, orbital emphysema, corneal ulcers, uveitis, and limitations of global motility due to entrapment by bone fragments may accompany orbital fractures.

☞ Orbital fractures can result in displacement of the globe and have the potential for globe penetrating bone fragments.

✓ Minor orbital rim fractures may not require surgical correction unless fracture fragments are impinging on the globe or perfect cosmesis is required.

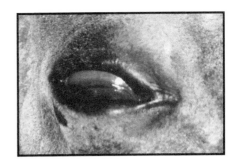

Figure 3-5 Change in globe position, eyelid swelling, and loss of orbital rim symmetry are present in a horse with an orbital fracture.

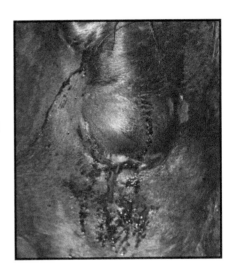

Figure 3-6 Severe periorbital swelling and drainage are present following trauma to the head.

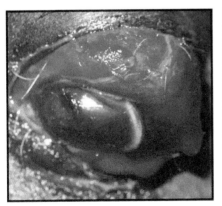
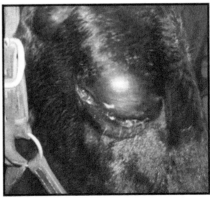

Figure 3-7 (left) Severe conjunctival swelling and a ruptured globe are present following head trauma.

Figure 3-8 (right) Lid swelling and discharge from orbital cellulitis following orbital trauma. (From Ann Dwyer).

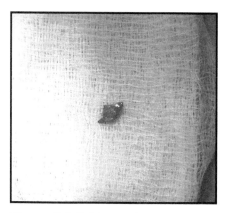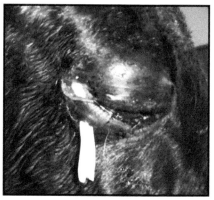

Figure 3-9 (left) Bone fragments were present in the horse in Figure 3-8. (From Ann Dwyer).

Figure 3-10 (right) A drain was used to treat the orbital cellulitis in the horse in Figure 3-8. (From Ann Dwyer).

Serious periorbital fractures should be surgically repaired quickly as fibrous union of the fractured pieces begins within one week following the injury to make elevation and realignment very difficult. Interosseous wiring with stainless steel suture, bone plating and cancellous bone grafts may be necessary to immobilize and repair extensive orbital fractures.

Foreign Bodies can lead to Orbital Abscesses

✓ Older horses tend to develop neoplasia, whereas foals and yearlings may be prone to acute orbital trauma and cellulitis/abscesses. Cellulitis may be associated with fever, blepharedema, swelling of the supraorbital fossa, nictitans protrusion, chemosis and corneal edema.

Head trauma can cause **globe proptosis**. Proptosis is forward displacement of the eye from the orbit. It is seen commonly with retrobulbar hemorrhage and edema following penetrating orbital trauma. In cases of traumatic globe proptosis, careful ophthalmic examination will dictate viability of the eye. Lack of an indirect pupillary reflex to the normal eye, and miosis with severe hypotony and hyphema indicates severe trauma and poor visual prognosis. Temporary tarsorrhaphy is recommended for proptosis.

Orbital Tumors

✓ Meningioma, neuroendocrine tumor, lipoma, adenocarcinoma, lymphoma, melanoma, sarcoid, squamous cell carcinoma, hemangiosarcoma, multilobular osteoma, medulloepithelioma, schwannoma, and neurofibroma have all been found in the equine orbit. (Figures 3-11 to 3-13) Orbital lymphoma can be focal and the tumor successfully removed surgically.

✓ Orbitotomy can be diagnostic and therapeutic, however it is a difficult surgery that may require orthopedic instruments.

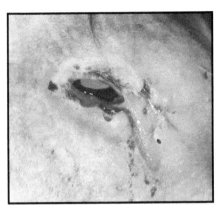 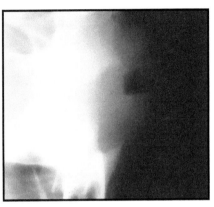

Figure 3-11 (left) Severe swelling of the periorbital region is present in this old Paint horse with a squamous cell carcinoma invading the bony orbit.

Figure 3-12 (right) A radiographic image of the horse in Figure 3-11 shows bony invasion of the orbit by the tumor at the outer edge of the image.

Figure 3-13 Orbital SCC causing purulent ocular discharge.

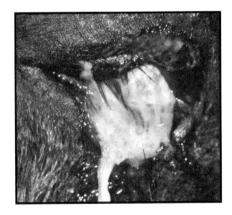

☞ Orbitotomy with tumor debulking and adjunctive therapy can be used in discrete orbital tumors of the horse. Exenteration and tumor debulking may be palliative in advanced tumors.

✓ Recurrence of retrobulbar tumors is possible after primary treatment depending on the definitive diagnosis.

Suture Line Periostitis

✓ Periostitis of the naso-frontal suture can cause profound periocular swelling, severe chemosis, and nasolacrimal duct obstruction in horses. Unilateral and bilateral cases are noted. The etiology is not understood but may be nutritional. Enlargement of the frontal bone suture lines can persist following systemic NSAID therapy.

Treatment of Equine Orbital Disease

✓ Treatment of orbital soft tissue trauma depends on the specific ocular area damaged, the degree of dysfunction or displacement, and the involvement of adjacent orbital tissues.

Orbital diseases, once identified, may be treated medically, as in minor trauma, or may need surgical attention (e.g. orbital neoplasia or fractures) (see Figures 3-6 to 3-10).

⚷ Systemically administered antibiotics and nonsteroidal anti-inflammatory agents are indicated to minimize infection and to reduce pain and eyelid swelling. Banamine or phenylbutazone can be given for pain associated with the orbital disease.

⚷ Systemic antibiotics should be administered in cases of trauma or suspected orbital infection. The globe itself may benefit from topical ophthalmic lubricants or antibiotics. Periorbital swelling can be alleviated by judicious use of nonsteroidal antiinflammatories.

⚷ Topically applied corticosteroids should be used only in the presence of an intact corneal epithelium. Dimethyl sulfoxide can be applied topically to edematous eyelids to reduce lid swelling.

⚷ **Enucleation** refers to surgical removal of the globe, conjunctiva and nictitating membrane. It is a painful procedure. The remaining orbital contents undergo severe atrophy and contraction such that the anophthalmic equine orbit exhibits severe pitting of the skin covering the orbit post-enucleation. Enucleation may be recommended to remove a painful, blind, diseased eye, and can be necessary for severe disease of the globe, adnexa, conjunctiva and nictitans.

General anesthesia is best for enucleating horses but a retrobulbar injection of anesthetic can aid recovery of horses having an eye enucleated. A transconjunctival injection of 6 cc lidocaine (20 mg/cc) and 6 cc bupivicaine (7.5 mg/cc) with a curved 3.5 inch 22 gauge needle till the globe nearly proptoses is satisfactory (Figures 3-14 and 3-15).

Standing enucleations with orbital nerve blocks can be attempted successfully in horses at anesthetic risk.

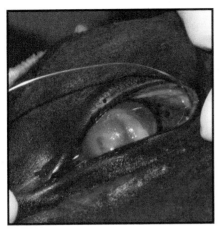 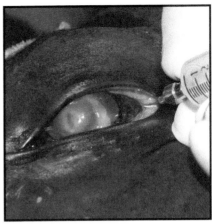

Figure 3-14 (left) A transconjunctival injection of 6 cc lidocaine (20mg/cc) and 6cc bupivicaine (7.5 mg/cc) with a curved 3,5 inch 22 gauge needle is used for orbital nerve blocks for enucleation. The needle is inserted through the lateral conjunctiva.

Figure 3-15 (right) The needle is inserted posteriorly and anesthetic injected until the globe begins to proptose.

✓ **Orbital exenteration** is a surgical technique used to remove malignant tumors of the orbit that are unresponsive to chemotherapy and/or radiotherapy. In this procedure the globe and entire orbital contents, including periorbita, are surgically removed.

✓ An **intra orbital prosthesis** may be placed in the orbit to replace the globe if risk of infection or tumor recurrence is low. A new type of orbital prosthesis minimizes the "pitting" following enucleation. (Figure 3-16) (Veterinary Ophthalmic Specialties, Moscow, ID; vos@vetospec.com; 208-882-9350) (Figures 3-17 to 3-19). Prostheses can be rejected (Figure 3-20).

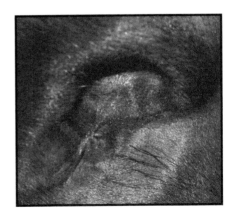

Figure 3-16 Severe pitting of the orbital socket follows enucleation in horses.

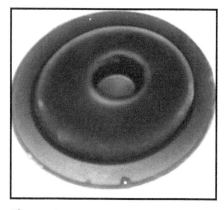
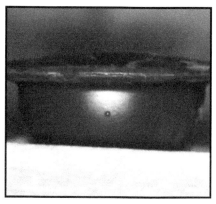

Figure 3-17 (left) New silicone orbital implant minimizes postenucleation socket pitting. The rounded side fits into the orbit.

Figure 3-18 (right) A side view of Figure 3-17 orbital implant.

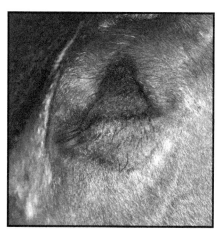

Figure 3-19 The implant in Figure 3-18 reduces the collapse of the skin over the orbital socket postenucleation.

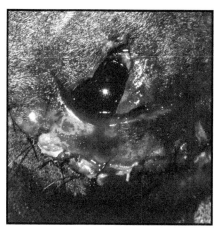

Figure 3-20 Exposure of the implant can occur if contamination of the orbit occurred preoperatively or intraoperately.

✓ The **intrascleral (ISP) or intraocular silicone prostheses** has been used in horses as a cosmetic alternative to enucleation. The ISP replaces the intraocular contents that are removed by evisceration. Implants of 38-44 mm in diameter are recommended for adult hoses, but should not be placed in eyes with severe corneal disease, intraocular neoplasia or infectious panophthalmitis (Figures 3-21 to 3-23).

✎ **Tarsorrhaphies** are beneficial to proptosed eyes and should not be removed until most of the periorbital swelling has subsided, usually 5 to 7 days.

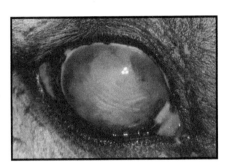

Figure 3-21 Appearance of the eye 2 years following placement of an intrascleral prosthesis for treatment of a painful blind eye due to equine recurrent uveitis in a Lipizanner stallion. (Preoperative image is Figure 7-81).

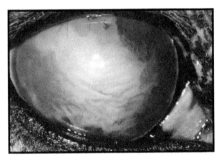
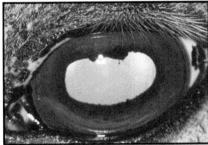

Figure 3-22 (left) The appearance seven years postoperatively in the horse in Figure 3-21.

Figure 3-23 (right) Normal eye of the horse in Figure 3-21.

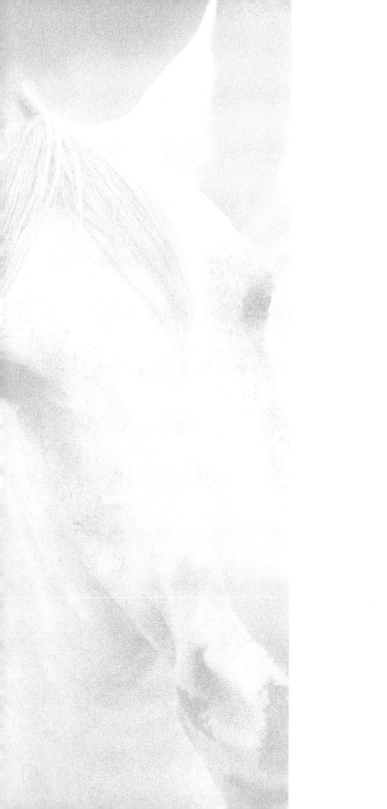

Section 4

The Eyelids, Conjunctiva and Lacrimal System

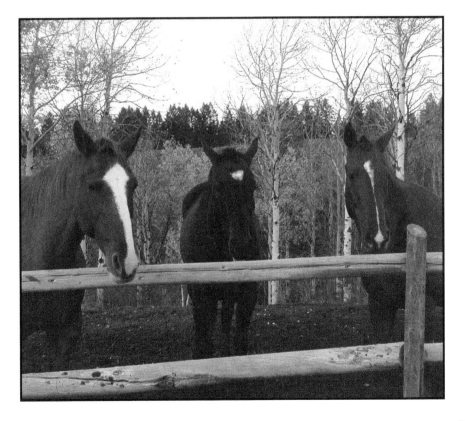

♥ Thin and highly vascularized, the eyelids contain muscles, connective tissue, cilia, glands that produce components of the tear film and a tarsal plate that gives the free edge of the lid support. They are lined with conjunctiva. The major issues that arise with eyelids are trauma, inflammation, and neoplasia. Occasionally lids can be malformed. Prompt, definitive therapy is needed when any condition threatens the anatomy or function of the lids. Eyelids can heal VERY well if surgery is done with careful technique.

Traumatic Eyelid Lacerations

Lid trauma needs to be corrected as soon and as accurately as possible to prevent undesirable scarring, entropion (Figures 4-1 to 4-4), ectropion (Figures 4-5 to 4-8), blepharitis, and secondary corneal desiccation and ulceration. Eyelids are highly vascular and have a great capacity to heal and resist infection. They can also swell quite dramatically in cases of blepharitis (Figures 4-9 to 4-11). Minimal debridement is needed due to their extensive blood supply, and an eyelid "tag" or pedicle flap should never be excised as exposure keratitis and corneal ulceration can result (Figures 4-12 and 4-13).

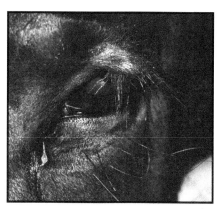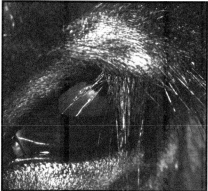

Figure 4-1 (left) Slight blepharospasm, entropion and drooping of the upper eyelashesd in a Thoroughbred gelding is noted.

Figure 4-2 (right) Closeup view of Figure 4-1.

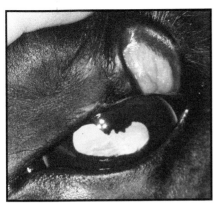 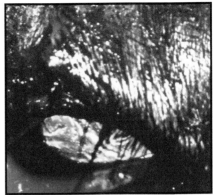

Figure 4-3 (left) Inversion of the upper lid due to malalignment of a lid laceration results in entropion in Figure 4-1.

Figure 4-4 (right) Surgical breakdown and eversion of this entropic lid was performed to restore lid margin integrity.

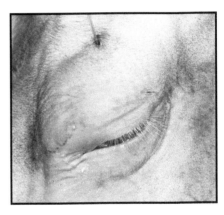

Figure 4-5 Upper eyelid swelling from cellulitis associated with a subpalpebral lavage system.

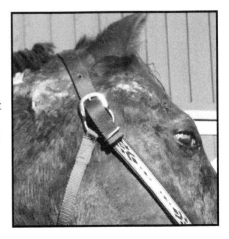

Figure 4-6 Retraction of forehead skin from a barn fire has caused cicatricial ectropion of the upper eyelid. Movement of the upper lid is still possible but not able to cover the entire cornea causing a chronic keratitis.
(Photo by Susan Gleason.)

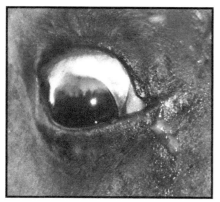
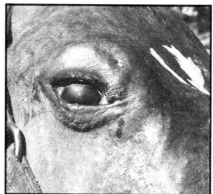

Figure 4-7 (left) Closeup of Figure 4-6. (Photo by Susan Gleason.)
Figure 4-8 (right) Releasing incisions in the forehead skin have reduced the ectropion. (Photo by Susan Gleason.)

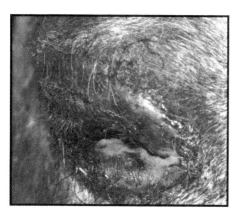

Figure 4-9 Severe blepharitis caused by a brush fire.

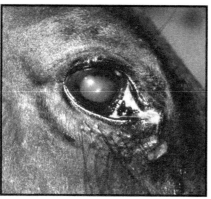
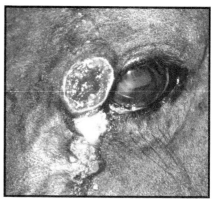

Figure 4-10 (left) Habronema blepharitis is bilateral in a Thoroughbred mare. The medial canthal lesions are typical.
Figure 4-11 (right) The other eye in the horse in Figure 4-10 has large erosive cutaneous lesions.

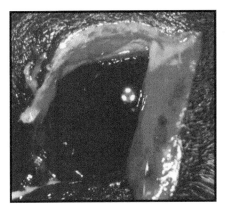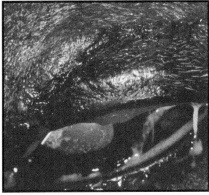

Figure 4-12 (left) A severe laceration of the upper lid has the lid margin remaining attached by a small pedicle.

Figure 4-13 (right) Surgical repair of the eyelid in Figure 4-12 successfully restored function to the lid.

✄ Upper eyelid damage is more significant in horses because the upper lid moves over more of the equine cornea than does the lower lid. Medial canthal lid trauma can involve the nasolacrimal system.

✄ THE MOST COMMON CAUSE OF LID LACERATION IS ENTRAPMENT OF THE LID IN A BUCKET HANDLE!!!

✓ It is important to thoroughly examine the globe both externally and via ophthalmoscopy. The nasolacrimal system should also be evaluated for damage when medial canthal injuries are present.

Preservation of the eyelid margin is critical if at all possible in order to preserve eyelid function (Figures 4-14 to 4-19).

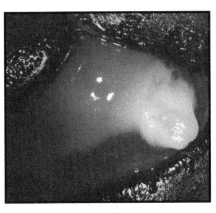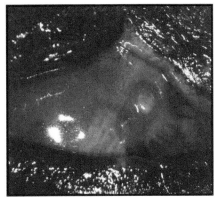

Figure 4-14 Corneal dessication from exposure keratitis caused by a upper eyelid defect resulted in a fungal ulcer.

Figure 4-15 The ulcer in the eye in Figure 4-14 is healed after three weeks of intensive medical therapy.

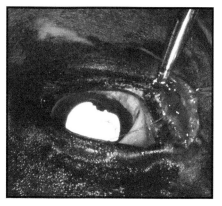 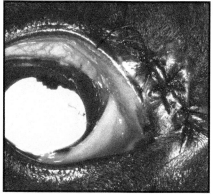

Figure 4-16 (left) A chronic eyelid laceration is present in this horse.
Figure 4-17 (right) The laceration in Figure 4-16 is sutured.

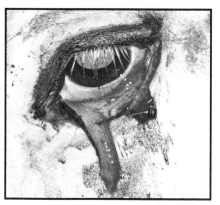 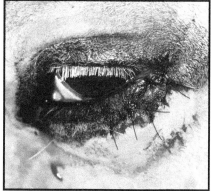

Figure 4-18 (left) Severe lower lid laceration requires surgical correction.
Figure 4-19 (right) The lid in Figure 4-18 three weeks postoperatively has healed nicely.

☞ The repaired lesion must be protected from "self-trauma" with fly masks or hard cups.

Basic principles of eyelid laceration surgery include:

1) First restore and align the eyelid margin and palpebral fissure.

2) Two-layer closure of the laceration is stronger than one layer.

3) Eyelid swelling may be such postoperatively that corneal protection is needed.

4) Postoperative care includes topical and/or systemic antibiotics, and a tetanus booster.

✓ Leeches may be used on reconstructed eyelid lacerations in cases suffering from severe swelling due to impaired venous circulation.

✓ **Blepharitis** may be associated with infection, trauma, foreign bodies, and neoplasia. The swelling can be pronounced. Blepharitis is generally treated with topical and systemic medications.

✓ **Onchocerciasis** can cause blepharitis, conjunctivitis, keratitis and uveitis. Treatment involves administration of systemic ivermectin and topical steroids. Granulomas may require debridement under sedation and topical anesthesia.

✓ **Meibomianitis** is characterized by "cheesy" abscesses of the meibomium glands of the tarsal plate. May affect all 4 lid margins; idiopathic in origin. Treatment involves incision of the gland conjunctiva with a #15 scalpel blade and curettage of the debris with a small curette. Inspissated material may be gritty. Post operative therapy includes topical and/or systemic antibiotics and corticosteroids. Recurrence is common.

Neoplasia of the Lids

✓ **Eyelid melanomas** are found in grey horses, with Arabians and Percherons also at increased risk. Melanomas may be single or multiple. Treatment is surgical excision and cryotherapy. Oral cimetidine (2.5-4.0 mg/kg TID) for two months has been recommended for cutaneous melanomas.

♥ **Sarcoids** are solitary or multiple tumors of the eyelids and periocular region of the horse (Figures 4-20 to 4-25).

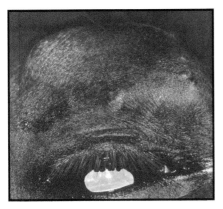 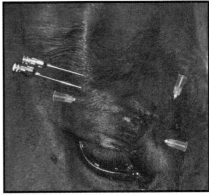

Figure 4-20 (left) A very large nodular sarcoid of the dorsal periorbital region.

Figure 4-21 (right) A series of intralesional cisplatin injections has reduced the size of the sarcoid in the horse in Figure 4-20.

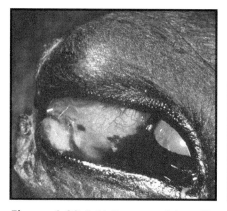
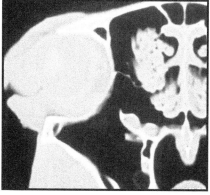

Figure 4-22 (left) Upper eyelid swelling caused by a sarcoid.
Figure 4-23 (right) CT finds the sarcoid mass in Figure 4-22 is compressing the globe but there is no skeletal involvement or sinus invasion.

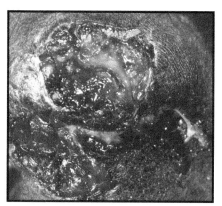
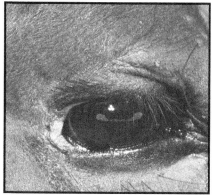

Figure 4-24 (left) Severe blepharitis following the fifth injection of BCG in the lesion of Figure 4-22.

Figure 4-25 (right) The sarcoid remains healed 9 months following therapy of the eye in Figure 4-22.

Retroviruses and papilloma viruses may be involved in the etiology. It is suspected that flies may be able to transfer sarcoid cells from one horse to traumatic skin lesions in other horses. There are geographic differences in the aggressiveness of the sarcoid in horses. Mules appear to suffer from an aggressive form of sarcoid. Lippizaners may be genetically resistant to sarcoids.

☗ The sarcoid lesion induces a fibrovascular inflammatory response that may mask the actual size of the sarcoid. Loss of muscle function occurs as the sarcoid invades eyelid muscles. The tumor cells are most prevalent near the rete pegs of the epithelium. They are rare in the large sarcoid "masses".

☙─⚔ Immunotherapy for sarcoids includes autogenous vaccines, and immunomodulators derived from mycobacterial products. The use of autogenous vaccines derived from sarcoid tumor homogenates, or cell-free tumor extracts has variable results. Immunomodulation using attenuated Mycobacterium bovis cell wall extracts such as the immunostimulant Bacillus Calmette-Gaérin (BCG), however, has produced reasonable remission rates. BCG alters sarcoid antigens such that they are recognized as foreign bymacrophages. Acid fast bacteria can be found in the sarcoids post-BCG injection.

☙─⚔ Shrinking the sarcoid lesion with antipsoriasis skin ointments and/or topical 5-fluorouracil (5-FU) for two weeks may be beneficial before using BCG. Topical 5% Imiquimod has been used QD for 8 days topically, then off 8 days, and repeated for another cycle for sarcoids. A lot of tissue swelling occurs.

✓ Surgical resection of necrotic tissue is controversial with some experts suggesting it will exacerbate the sarcoid.

☙─⚔ Cryotherapy, hyperthermia, carbon dioxide laser excision, intralesional chemotherapy, and intralesional radiotherapy can also be effective for sarcoid.

✓ Intralesional chemotherapeutics including 5-FU or cisplatin have been used with varying success rates.

✓ Interferon has been used systemically for very large, aggressive equine sarcoids.

✓ Homeopathic ointments (eg. bloodroot based pastes) such as XXTERRA® and caustic chemical lotions are effective in some sarcoids.

☙─⚔ **Mast cell tumors** may mimic habronemiasis and are associated with eosinophilic invasion of the lid.

♥ **Squamous cell carcinoma (SCC)** is the most common tumor of the eye and adnexa in horses (Figures 4-26 to 4-37). The etiopathogenesis may be related to the ultraviolet (UV) component of solar radiation, periocular pigmentation, and an increased susceptibility to carcinogenesis. The UV component is the most plausible carcinogenic agent associated with SCC, as it targets the tumor suppressor gene p53, which is altered in equine SCC.

● SCC may invade the periocular soft tissues, bony rim of the orbit, sinuses, brain, and metastasize to regional lymph nodes, salivary glands and lungs. Guttural pouch lymph nodes on the side of the SCC should be carefully examined. Rates of metastasis approach 18% in some studies. Tumor recurrence is highest in cases only treated with surgery. Diagnosis is based on biopsy, cytology, location, appearance, breed, and age of the horse.

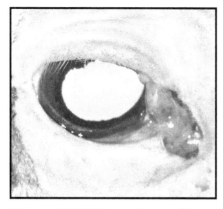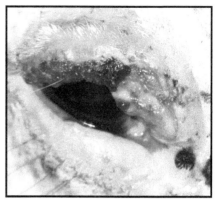

Figure 4-26 (left) Invasive, medial canthal, eyelid squamous cell carcinoma.
Figure 4-27 (right) Very invasive SCC of upper lid.

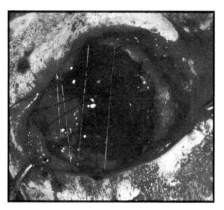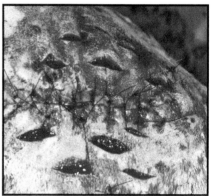

Figure 4-28 (left) Enucleation of the globe and forehead skin was used for treatment of Figure 4-27. A layer of nonabsorbable sutures is used to form a mesh over the orbital opening to minimize pitting of the overlying skin.
Figure 4-29 (right) Releasing incisions allow forward movement of skin to cover the opening of the orbit in the horse in Figure 4-27.

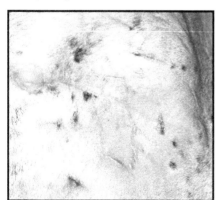

Figure 4-30 The horse remains SCC-free six months postoperatively in the horse in Figure 4-27.

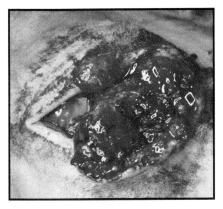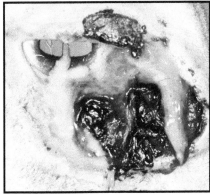

Figure 4-31 (left) A large and invasive eyelid SCC in a white horse.
Figure 4-32 (right) SCC necrosis is evident 2 weeks following intralesional Cisplatin in Figure 4-31.

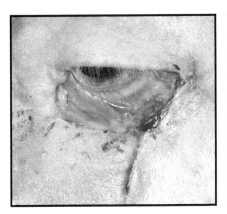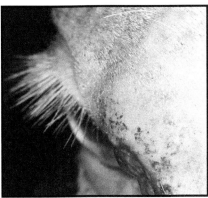

Figure 4-33 (left) Surgery and Cisplatin treatment resolved the SCC in Figure 4-31. There is some conjunctival irritation associated lower lid ectropion.
Figure 4-34 (right) Large SCC of the medial upper eyelid in this Paint.

Figure 4-35 Intralesional Cisplatin and ND-YAG laser therapy were used to treat the SCC in Figure 4-34. The laser burns are evident.

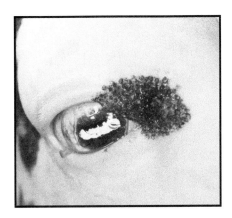

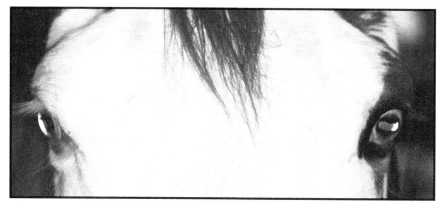

Figure 4-36 The SCC in Figure 4-34 is not evident three months following therapy.

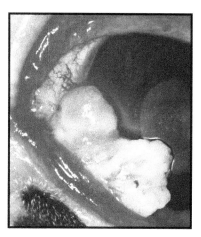

Figure 4-37 Proliferative squamous cell carcinoma is present in this white horse.

✓ Prevalence in horses increases with age with the mean age at diagnosis 11.1 ± 0.4 years in one report.

✓ Belgians, Clydesdales and other draft horses have a high prevalence of ocular SCC, followed by Appaloosas and Paints, with the least prevalence found in Arabians, Thoroughbreds and Quarterhorses.

✓ White, grey-white, and palomino hair colors predispose to ocular SCC, with less prevalence in bay, brown and black hair coats (Figure 4-38).

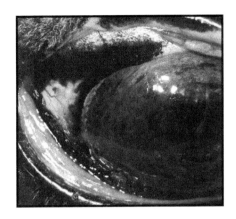

Figure 4-38 Conjunctival vitiligo or depigmentation may predispose to squamous cell carcinoma.

☞ Cryotherapy, immunotherapy, irradiation, radio-frequency hyperthermia, CO_2 laser ablation, or intralesional chemotherapy should follow surgical excision of equine ocular SCC. Additionally, reconstructive eyelid surgery may be required when eyelid margins are lost following tumor excision, and conjunctival grafts are indicated following keratectomy for corneal SCC (see Figures 4-31 to 4-36).

✓ Immunotherapy with Bacillus Calmette-Gaérin (BCG) cell wall extract has been used successfully for large periocular SCC in horses.

✓ Piroxicam (Feldene; 150 mg PO SID for 3 months, then reduce) is a COX2 inhibitor and may slow growth of unoperable SCC as prostaglandins may induce tumor growth in horses.

✓ Chemotherapy of invasive eyelid SCC with intralesional, slow release cisplatin has been used with and without surgical debulking (see Figures 4-31 and 4-32) and (Figure 4-39).

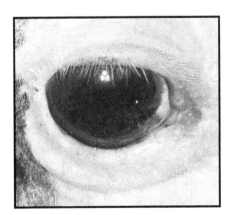

Figure 4-39 Intralesional cisplatin has reduced the size of the tumor in the horse in Figure 4-26.

✓ Topical 5-fluorouracil (1% 5-FU TID), or 0.01 to 0.04% mitomycin C (MMC, QID) is effective for corneal SCC in situ, and may be beneficial for extensive periocular SCC.

☛ Tumors may be removed by surgical excision alone if adequate margins can be obtained. However, adjunctive therapy is often recommended to improve the chance for a complete cure, especially with large or invasive tumors.

✓ Small, superficial tumors may be treated with radio-frequency hyperthermia or cryosurgery. Malignant cells are killed with local temperatures of 41 to 50 degrees C, following surgical excision.

✓ Cryosurgery with liquid nitrogen or nitrous oxide induces cryonecrosis of malignant cells when temperatures of -20 to -40 degrees C are achieved using a double freeze-thaw technique.

✓ Excision of corneal limbal SCC followed by CO_2 laser ablation has also been advocated.

✓ Radiotherapy with beta irradiation (strontium 90) is very beneficial in superficial SCC of the cornea and limbus following superficial keratectomy.

☛ Brachytherapy using cesium 137, radon 222, cobalt 60, or iridium 192 may be employed following surgical debulking of invasive eyelid tumors. Interstitial radiation therapy has the advantage of providing continuous exposure of the tumor to high levels of radiation over a period of time.

The Conjunctiva

✓ Conjunctivitis is inflammation of the mucous membrane that covers the posterior aspects of the eyelids (palpebral conjunctiva), the nictitans, and the sclera (bulbar conjunctiva) (Figure 4-40). It is a nonspecific finding that indicates ocular inflammation, and may also be seen in systemic disease (Figure 4-41). Infectious and noninfectious diseases of the lids, cornea, sclera, anterior uvea, nasolacrimal system, and orbit can result in conjunctivitis. The conjunctiva is a mucous membrane that can reflect systemic dysfunction through color changes, as in anemia and jaundice. Neoplasia may involve the conjunctiva.

♥ THE EYE GETS RED OR HAS CONJUNCTIVITIS IN NEARLY ALL TYPES OF EYE DISEASE. THE EYE HAS LIMITED WAYS TO REACT TO INJURY!

✓ *Dermoids (choristoma) are generally pigmented in horses and may have hair follicle development. They are reported to occur on the conjunctiva and cornea of foals.*

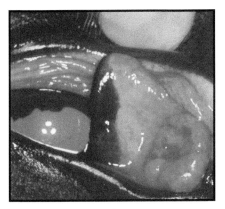 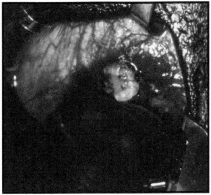

Figure 4-40 (left) This horse has lymphoid hyperplasia and conjunctivitis of the third eyelid due to environmental irritants.

Figure 4-41 (right) A white focal carcinoma in situ is found in the lateral conjunctiva near the limbus in this darkly pigmented thoroughbred mare.

♥ **Squamous cell carcinoma** is the most common tumor affecting the equine conjunctiva and can masquerade as simple conjunctivitis in the early stages. The prevalence increases with age, (see Figure 4-37) and (Figure 4-42).

Conjunctival lymphoma can masquerade or appear as conjunctivitis. It may be estrogen responsive and appear with ovarian tumors (Figure 4-42).

✓ **Habronemiasis** is a parasitic disease resulting in conjunctival and ocular granulomas. Onchocerciasis is a parasitic disease which can cause inflammation of the conjunctiva, cornea, and anterior uvea (Figures 4-10, 4-11, 4-43 and 4-44). Flareups of uveitis may occur following therapy for onchocerciasis. Thelazia lacrymalis is a commensal parasite of the conjunctival fornices and nasolacrimal ducts of horses, and can incite conjunctivitis, superficial keratitis, dacryocystitis, and mild eyelid swelling.

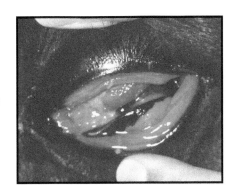

Figure 4-42 Conjunctival lymphoma masquerades as a severe conjunctivitis in this horse.

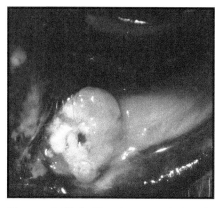 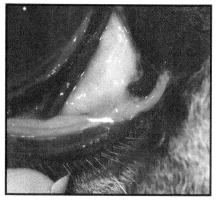

Figure 4-43 (left) Habronema induced conjunctival granulona of the nictitaus.
Figure 4-44 (right) Habronema granuloma mimics a third eyelind neoplasm.

✓ **Foal conjunctivitis** is associated with neonatal maladjustment syndrome, septicemia, immune-mediated hemolytic anemia, environmental allergens and irritants, dermoids, and subconjunctival or episcleral hemorrhages secondary to birth trauma.

✓ Conjunctivitis secondary to pneumonia is seen most commonly in 1 to 6 month old foals.

✓ Conjunctival hyperemia, chemosis (edema of the conjunctiva), ocular discharge that is serous (viral, allergic) to purulent (bacterial), and lymphoid follicle formation can be found in conjunctivitis.

♥ Conjunctivitis can be secondary to dacryocystitis, corneal stromal abscesses, corneal ulcers and uveitis. It can be found with environmental causes, and systemic diseases. Management of conjunctivitis due to an obstructed nasolacrimal duct may require surgical intervention.

✓ Icterus may be easily noticed in the conjunctiva (Figure 4-45).

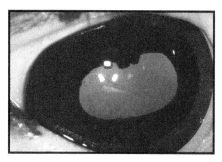

Figure 4-45 Icterus may be easily seen in the conjunctiva.

☛ Complete ophthalmic examination is indicated to identify adnexal and ocular causes of conjunctivitis. Thorough adnexal exam, fluorescein staining to identify the presence of corneal ulcers, and examination for signs of anterior uveitis (aqueous flare, miosis, hypotony) are important. Examination behind the nictitans may reveal a foreign body or debris. Consider cannulation and flushing of the nasolacrimal duct to rule out nasolacrimal disease. If conjunctival laceration with hypotony and/or hyphema is present, rule out scleral laceration.

☛ **Bacterial conjunctivitis** is treated with topical a broad-spectrum antibiotic initially (triple antibiotic is usually appropriate), which may change after results of bacterial culture and sensitivity are available. Treat every 6 hours to 12 hours depending on severity of disease. Topical corticosteroids are indicated following resolution of the infection.

☛ Infectious conjunctivitis usually responds to appropriate treatment. Failure to respond or recurrence suggests an unidentified underlying cause (i.e., recurrent bacterial conjunctivitis associated with an unrecognized foreign body). Course and prognosis of conjunctival neoplasia depends on the specific type of neoplasia and the extent of invasion of surrounding tissues.

✓ **Allergic conjunctivitis** is treated with topical corticosteroids and is often difficult to eliminate completely due to the nature of the horse's environment. The prognosis associated with conjunctivitis secondary to systemic or complicated ocular disease varies with the specific disease. Eosinophils may invade the conjunctiva in several conditions (Figures 4-46 and 4-47).

☛ **Treatment of conjunctival neoplasia** may involve local resection, with adjunctive beta-irradiation, brachytherapy, cryotherapy, radiofrequency hyperthermia, or intralesional chemotherapy. Topical 1% 5 FU QD for one week, then BID for one week, no therapy for the third week, QD again for the fourth week, and then BID for the fifth week may aid treatment of equine conjunctival lymphoma. Enucleation or exenteration may be necessary depending on the type of conjunctival neoplasia and extent of invasion.

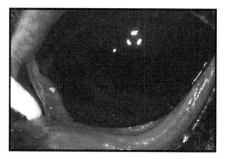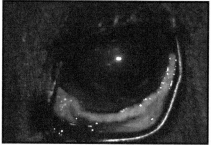

Figure 4-46 (left) Eosinophils infiltrate the conjunctiva covering this nictitans.
Figure 4-47 (right) Eosinophil invasion of the conjunctiva causes thickening of the nictitans in this eye.

Nictitans

✓ The nictitating membrane, nictitans, or third eyelid (TE) consists of a T-shaped cartilage with a seromucoid gland located at its base. The nictitans is covered on both the palpebral and bulbar surfaces with conjunctiva, and diseases affecting the conjunctiva can also involve the nictitans (see Figure 1-1), (Figures 4-48 and 4-49). Inflammation of the TE conjunctiva alone suggests neoplasia, parasites, or nasolacrimal duct obstruction.

✓ Movement of the nictitans is nearly horizontal from nasal to lateral in horses, It distributes the tear film and protects the cornea.

✓ Protrusion of the nictitating membrane is usually a nonspecific sign of ocular pain. TE protrusion in such cases is passive and occurs due to retraction of the globe by the retractor bulbi muscle.

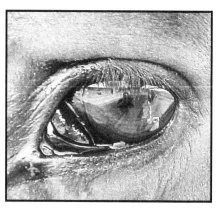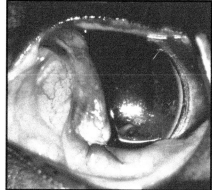

Figure 4-48 (left) The nictitans is prominent in this 4 year old Andalusian mare.
Figure 4-49 (right) The nictitans cartilage is deformed causing a scrolled appearance to this nictitans.

♥ A reduction in globe size or orbital contents can result in nictitans protrusion (see Figures 2-58 and 2-60).

✓ Systemic diseases can also cause nictitans protrusion due to enophthalmos from a reduction in orbital contents, or exophthalmos from an increase in orbital contents.

✓ **Horner's syndrome** is a loss of sympathetic innervation to the globe and TE, and can be a result of central, preganglionic, or postganglionic sympathetic lesions.

✓ Horner's syndrome signs in horses include ptosis, nictitans protrusion, slight miosis, hyperemia of the nasal and conjunctival mucosa, and increased temperature and sweating of the base of the ear, side of face, and neck of the affected side.

✓ **Hyperkalemic periodic paralysis** is seen most commonly in Quarter Horses and can cause protrusion of the nictitans.

✓ **Squamous cell carcinoma**, the most common neoplasm affecting the equine nictitans, has a high prevalence in draft horses, Appaloosas, and Paints (Figure 4-50).

♥ **Tetanus** causes bilateral protrusion and rapid movement ("flashing") of the nictitans, spasms of the masseter muscles, stiff gait, and increased sensitivity to external stimulation.

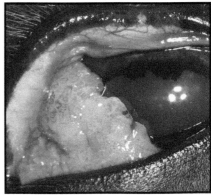

Figure 4-50 Squamous cell carcinoma of the nictitans is present in this horse.

The Nasolacrimal System

✓ The nasolacrimal system has both secretory and drainage components. The lacrimal and nictitans glands, the meibomian glands, and the conjunctival goblet cells produce the tear film. Tears drain through the upper and lower eyelid puncta at the medial canthus into the nasolacrimal canaliculi, and subsequently to the nasolacrimal sac. Tears then move from the nasolacrimal sac into the nasolacrimal duct, a portion of which is contained in the lacrimal bone of the maxilla. (see Figure 2-10) The nasolacrimal duct opens at the nasal punctum located at the mucocutaneous junction of the ventrolateral portion of the floor of the nasal vestibule.

Keratoconjunctivitis Sicca (KCS)

KCS or "dry eye" in horses is a group of clinical signs related to a lack of tears. Corneal ulcers, corneal pigmentation, conjunctivitis and blepharospasm may be seen. The Schirmer tear test values (normal is 14-34-mm wetting/minute) are less than 10-mm wetting/minute in horses with KCS (Figures 4-51 to 4-54). The tear film breakup time will be <10 seconds in many horse with KCS although the Schirmer may be normal indicating a qualitative KCS.

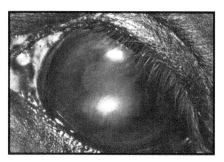 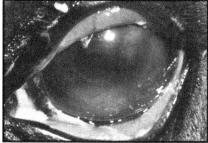

Figure 4-51 (left) This horse with KCS has a dry appearing cornea and a Schirmer tear test value of 2 mm wetting/minute. (From Sheila Crispin)

Figure 4-52 (right) This horse with KCS has a dry appearing cornea, red conjunctiva and a Schirmer tear test value of 6 mm wetting/minute. (From Sheila Crispin)

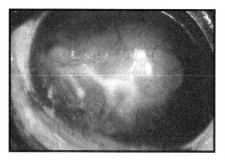 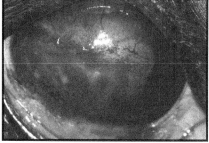

Figure 4-53 (left) Slight fluorescein dye retention is present over a scarred cornea in a horse with KCS.

Figure 4-54 (right) A large area of Rose bengal dye retention indicates tear film instability in the horse with KCS in Figure 4-53.

✓ Parasympathetic stimulation of the lacrimal gland causes release of tears. Fractures of the stylohyoid bone or proximal part of the vertical ramus of the mandible damage the superficial petrosal nerve that contains the lacrimal gland parasympathetic innervation to cause KCS. Due to the anatomical proximity of cranial nerve VII to the lacrimal gland innervation, facial palsy may also be present.

✓ KCS may also be evident in some cases of vestibular disease and in temporohyoid osteoarthropathy (middle ear disease) of horses.

✓ KCS associated with mucin layer instability appears common in horses.

✓ In the USA, KCS has been associated with locoweed poisoning, and KCS from eosinophilic keratoconjunctivitis causing dacryoadenitis.

✓ Treatment is palliative in many cases and consists of topical artificial tears and cyclosporine A. The prognosis for recovery of tear production is generally guarded.

Dacryocystitis

✓ Dacryocystitis is inflammation of the lacrimal sac and nasolacrimal duct, and is seen frequently in horses (see Figure 2-49) and (Figure 4-55).

☞ Dacryocystitis may develop as a primary problem or be secondary to duct obstruction. Eyelid puncta atresia, nasolacrimal duct agenesis, and nasal puncta atresia are congenital abnormalities that can result in severe dacryocystitis (see Figures 2-49 to 2-53). There are many potential causes of acquired obstruction of the nasolacrimal system (fractures, foreign bodies, neoplasia, granulomas, sinusitis), although often an underlying cause cannot be determined.

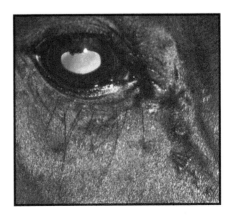

Figure 4-55 Dacryocystitis has scarred the skin near the medial canthus in this horse.

☙ Dacryocystitis associated with a congenital abnormality of the nasolacrimal system is usually seen within the first 3 to 4 months of life, and occasionally not until 1 to 2 years of age. Infection is usually present (see Figures 2-49 to 2-53).

☙ Thick mucopurulent discharge at the medial canthus, reflux exudation upon manipulation of the medial eyelid, and mild conjunctival hyperemia may be unilateral or bilateral when associated with congenital abnormalities of the nasolacrimal system. **Atresia of the nasal puncta** is most commonly unilateral. The globe and conjunctiva are usually not involved, unless chronic dacryocystitis has resulted in severe blepharoconjunctivitis (see Figures 2-49 to 2-53) and (Figures 4-56 to 4-58).

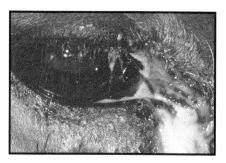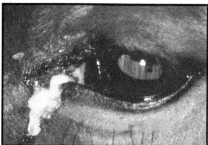

Figure 4-56 (left) Severe purulent discharge in a yearling with nasolacrimal duct agenesis and nasal puncta atresia.

Figure 4-57 (right) Discharge is also present to a lesser degree in the other eye of the horse in Figure 4-56.

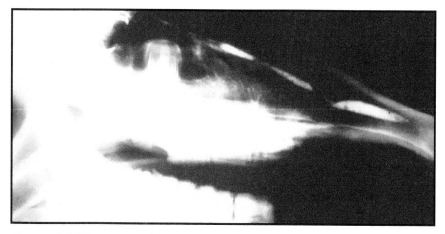

Figure 4-58 Dacryocystorhinogram of the horse in Figures 4-56 and 4-57 demonstrates radiopaque dye obstruction at the distal part of the nasolacrimal duct (right side of photo).

☞ It is important to differentiate dacryocystitis from other causes of mucopurulent ocular discharge including bacterial or parasitic conjunctivitis, neoplasia of eyelid or conjunctiva, secondary infection of globe or eyelid injury, and ocular foreign body.

♥ Complete ophthalmic examination is indicated to identify any primary ocular problem causing a mucopurulent discharge or secondary ocular involvement. Patency of the duct may be assessed initially by the fluorescein dye passage test (Figure 4-59). Fluorescein dye is instilled into the eye, and the nasal puncta is observed for appearance of fluorescein within 5 minutes. Attempts should be made to flush the duct with saline or irrigating solution from the patent puncta. Topical anesthetic should be applied to both the nasal mucosa and conjunctiva near the openings prior to flushing. Cannulation of the nasolacrimal duct is performed in congenital, chronic, or obstructed cases using a #5 French urinary catheter or polyethylene tubing (size 160) inserted through the nasal or eyelid puncta. The catheter may appear to hit a blind end several centimeters from the nasal opening and should be redirected laterally (Figure 4-60).

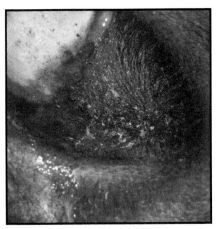 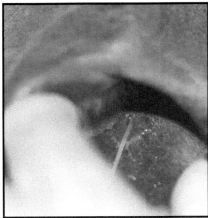

Figure 4-59 (left) Fluorescein drains from the nose indicating a patent nasolacrimal duct.

Figure 4-60 (right) The nasolacrimal duct opening in the nasal meatus is catheterized.

✔ Dental and oral examination should be performed if dental disease is suspected as the inciting cause of dacryocystitis.

♥ Aerobic and anaerobic bacterial culture and sensitivity of material flushed from the puncta and duct are beneficial in identifying the cause of persistent dacryocystitis. Systemic antibiotics but not topical antibiotics penetrate the nasolacrimal duct.

✔ Skull radiographs are valuable if a fracture is suspected from the history or physical exam. Contrast dacryocystorhinography is essential and assists in identifying the cause and location of the obstruction. It involves instillation of 4-6 ml of radiopaque solution into the puncta followed by plane film radiography.

☞ **Treatment of nasolacrimal puncta and duct agenesis** requires surgery(see Figures 2-49 to 2-53). Nasal puncta atresia necessitates surgical creation of a distal nasolacrimal duct opening in the nasal meatus. Flushing of the nasolacrimal system from the eyelid puncta results in dilation of nasal mucosal tissue overlying the site of the atretic puncta. This may be difficult to identify. A #5 French urinary catheter may be inserted at the eyelid puncta and gentle palpation utilized to feel the end of the catheter beneath the mucosa. A metal stylet (22 gauge surgical steel) inserted in the catheter can aid identification of the catheter end under the mucosa. This may be quite dorsal in the nasal meatus. A small endoscope or otoscope may aid visualization. An incision through the tissue over the catheter will establish patency. Placing the #5 French urinary catheter stent in the nasolacrimal duct will allow epithelialization of new puncta. Severe hemorrhage may occur following incision over the atretic nasal puncta and the area should be packed with gauze prior to surgery. The catheter is flushed with dilute betadine. Ends of the stent are sutured to the skin of the muzzle and near the medial canthus. The stent is left in place for 4 to 8 weeks. Systemic antibiotics and drainage around the stent speed healing of the dacryocystitis.

✔ Acquired obstructions are treated by removal of inciting cause when possible, irrigating the duct, and catheterization of the duct for 2 to 3 weeks. The indwelling stent catheter is sutured to the skin as described for congenital lesions. Systemic antibiotics are necessary for penetration into the infected tissue.

⊶ Acquired obstructions resulting in dacryocystitis are often more difficult to treat than congenital abnormalities. Foreign body and periodontal causes have the best response to therapy of acquired obstructions. Cannulation of the duct may be impossible in cases of neoplasia and maxillary fractures, and permanent correction of the obstruction and subsequent dacryocystitis may not be possible.

✓ Conjunctivorhinostomy involves creation of a mucous membrane-lined fistula between the lacrimal lake and nasal cavity. This procedure is indicated for nasolacrimal duct obstruction that cannot be relieved with flushing or cannulation.

Section 5

Corneal Ulceration

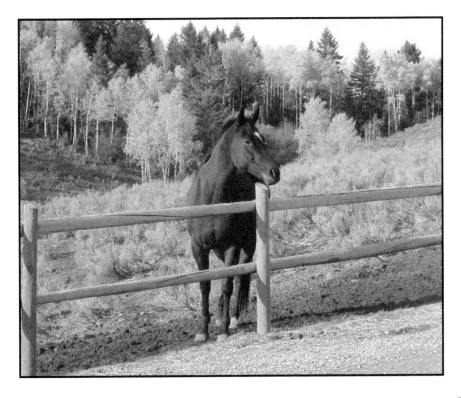

Corneal Ulceration

♥ Equine corneal ulceration is very common in horses and is a sight threatening disease requiring early clinical diagnosis, laboratory confirmation, and appropriate medical and surgical therapy.

✓ Ulcers can range from simple, superficial breaks or abrasions in the corneal epithelium, to full-thickness corneal perforations with iris prolapse (Figures 5-1 to 5-148).

✓ The prominent eye of the horse may predispose to traumatic corneal injury.

♠ Both bacterial and fungal keratitis in horses may present with a mild, early clinical course, but require prompt therapy if serious ocular complications are to be avoided.

♥ Corneal ulcers in horses should be aggressively treated no matter how small or superficial they may be. Corneal infection and iridocyclitis are always major concerns for even the slightest corneal ulcerations. Iridocyclitis or uveitis is present in all types of corneal ulcers and must be treated in order to preserve vision (see Figures 5-6, 5-7, 5-52, 5-56, 5-71, 5-91, and 5-94).

✓ Globe rupture, phthisis bulbi, and blindness are possible sequelae to corneal ulceration in horses (see Figure 5-144).

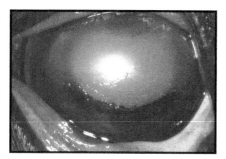 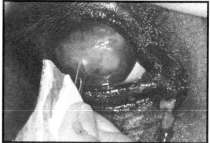

Figure 5-1 (left) A large, superficial fungal ulcer has a dry appearance.

Figure 5-2 (right) Three weeks later, cytology samples are again obtained with the handle end of a scalpel blade from the cornea in the horse in Figure 5-1. Profound granulation of the cornea is present after treatment for three weeks as the ulcer heals.

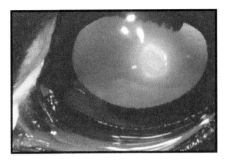 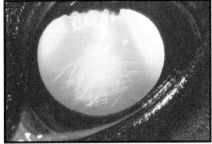

Figure 5-3 (left) A superficial ulcer stains with fluorescein dye.

Figure 5-4 (right) Following medical therapy and grid keratotomy, 20 days later the ulcer in Figure 5-3 has healed. Linear opacities in the cornea highlighted by the camera flash illumination are a result of the grid keratotomy.

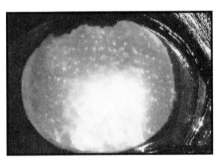 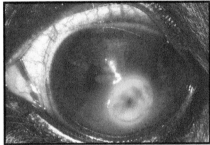

Figure 5-5 (left) Small dots are scars that resulted from the use of punctate keratotomy for an indolent ulcer.

Figure 5-6 (right) Axial corneal ulcer in Figure 5-5 has the gelatinous appearance of stromal melting. The center of the ulcer is thinner and has a dark appearance. The miotic pupil indicates uveitis.

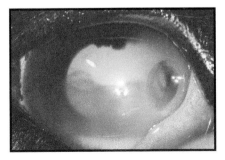 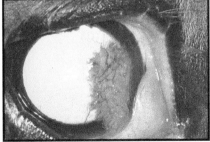

Figure 5-7 (left) Deep ulcer near the limbus with uveitis causing hypopyon ventrally and fibrin in the pupil.

Figure 5-8 (right) Three weeks postoperatively, a conjunctival flap is covering the ulcer in Figure 5-7. The signs of uveitis are absent.

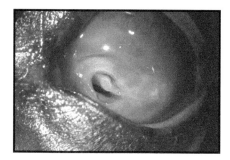
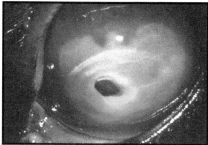

Figure 5-9 (left) Large diameter descemetocele indicates corneal rupture could occur.

Figure 5-10 (right) Descemetocele in Figure 5-9 has fluorescein retention at the edge of the lesion. Descemet's membrane does not stain with fluorescein.

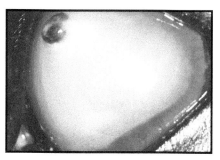
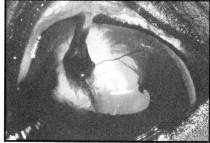

Figure 5-11 (left) Iris prolapse with corneal abscessation surrounding the prolapse, and severe hypopyon.

Figure 5-12 (right) The conjunctival flap repair of the cornea of the horse in Figure 5-11 is pigmented with some corneal scarring, and anterior and posterior synechia present 6.5 months postoperatively.

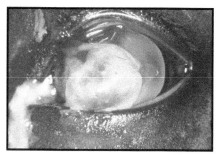
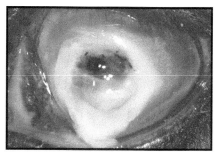

Figure 5-13 (left) The protruding iris is encased in fibrin in this severe iris prolapse caused by a large corneal laceration. There was no indirect pupillary light reflex or dazzle reflex and the eye was enucleated.

Figure 5-14 (right) Darkly pigmented iris protrudes from a melting necrotic cornea. There was no indirect pupillary light reflex or dazzle reflex and the eye was enucleated.

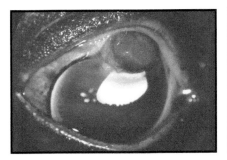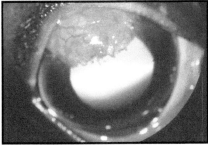

Figure 5-15 (left) Iris protrudes from a limbal laceration. The pupil is small and the anterior chamber is shallow.

Figure 5-16 (right) Mydriasis and a conjunctival flap over the perforating limbal lesion two days postoperatively in the horse in Figure 5-15.

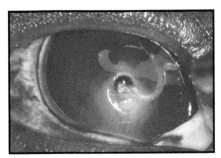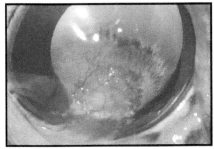

Figure 5-17 (left) Iris plugs the ruptured descemetocele in this horse. Miosis is present. It was repaired with a corneal transplant and conjunctival pedicle graft.

Figure 5-18 (right) Corneal vascularization is present near the surgical site 19 days postoperatively in the horse in Figure 5-17. Uveitis is absent.

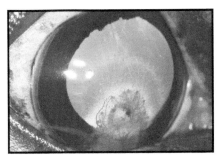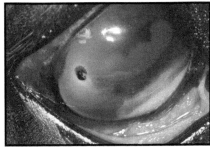

Figure 5-19 (left) Vascularization of the cornea and graft is reduced 35 days postoperatively in the horse in Figure 5-17.

Figure 5-20 (right) A small descemetocele is associated with hypopyon.

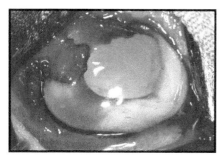
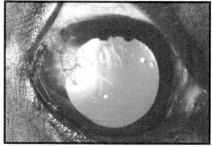

Figure 5-21 (left) Intraoperative photograph of a conjunctival pedicle graft used for treatment of the descemetocele in Figure 5-20.

Figure 5-22 (right) The conjunctival pedicle graft has speeded healing of the lesion in Figure 5-21 one month after surgery.

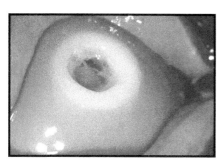
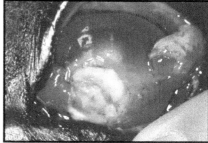

Figure 5-23 (left) White cellular infiltrate surrounds this descemetocele.

Figure 5-24 (right) Severe collagenolysis associated with a beta hemolytic Streptococcus infection has resulted in enzymatic destruction of a conjunctival bipedicle graft and exposure of the diseased ulcer site.

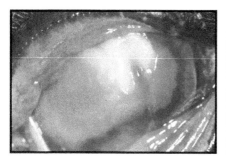
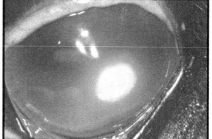

Figure 5-25 (left) Extensive corneal melting and necrosis caused by a beta hemolytic Streptococcus infection following a keratectomy for corneal tumor removal.

Figure 5-26 (right) Small fluorescein stained corneal ulcer with slight melting.

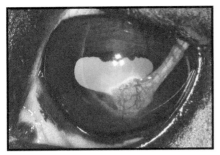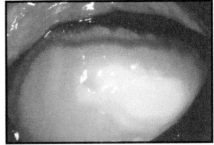

Figure 5-27 (left) A conjunctival pedicle graft over the ulcer in Figure 5-26 has healed the lesion.

Figure 5-28 (right) A large area of yellowish necrotic tissue indicates collagen breakdown from elevated tear film enzymatic activity due to a fungal infection.

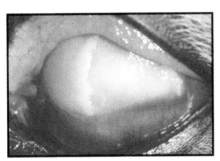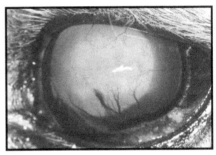

Figure 5-29 (left) Severe melting associated with this fungal ulcer. Note the clearing of the cornea as the limbal blood vessels move into the diseased area.

Figure 5-30 (right) Central corneal scarring and vascularization of the fungal ulcer in Figure 5-29 is present after 3 weeks of medical therapy. The uveitis is absent.

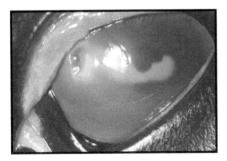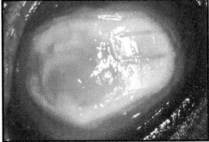

Figure 5-31 (left) Severe melting of an ulcer is noted in this horse.

Figure 5-32 (right) The lines in the necrotic yellow portion of this fungal ulcer are from a grid keratotomy. Grid keratotomies should only be performed in superficial, non infected ulcers.

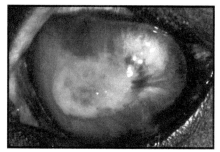

Figure 5-33 Granulation tissue covers the fungal ulcer that received inappropriate grid keratotomy in Figure 5-32 one month later.

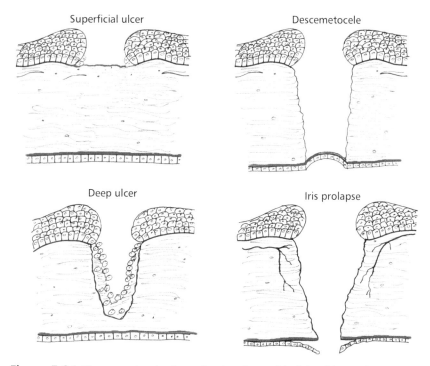

Superficial ulcer   Descemetocele

Deep ulcer   Iris prolapse

Figure 5-34 Ulcers can involve loss of only a few epithelial cell layers (micro-erosions) or the entire epithelium is absent (superficial ulcers); the epithelium and some stroma are missing (deep ulcers); the entire stroma can be lost (descemetocele); or an ulcer can result in rupture of the cornea to cause iris prolapse.

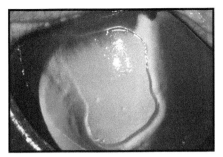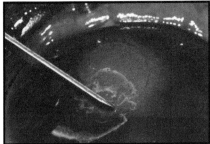

Figure 5-35 (left) A nonhealing, superficial erosion has only slight dorsal vascularization.

Figure 5-36 (right) A 20 gauge needle is used to debride a noninfectious superficial ulcer.

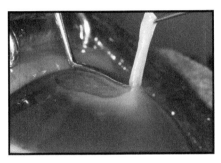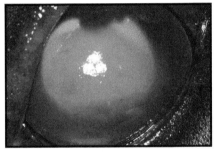

Figure 5-37 (left) A corneal dissector is used for a keratectomy to remove loose, abnormal epithelium in a nonhealing corneal ulcer.

Figure 5-38 (right) Rose Bengal staining indicates tear film instability in a horse with corneal edema.

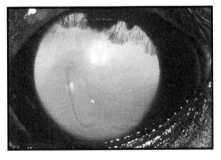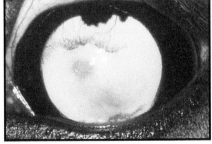

Figure 5-39 (left) The edematous epithelium sloughs off to reveal an ulcer one week later in the horse from Figure 5-38.

Figure 5-40 (right) The superficial ulcer is smaller with some vascularization of the cornea one week after Figure 5-39.

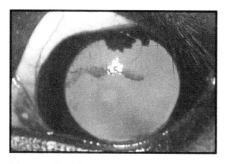
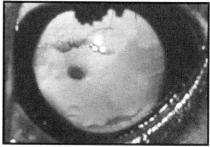

Figure 5-41 (left) Fluorescein staining of the eye.
Figure 5-42 (right) Rose Bengal staining of the eye in Figure 5-41. The tear film is not stable over the bare corneal stroma which can lead to slow healing.

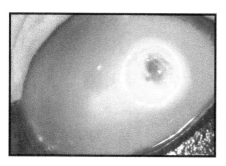
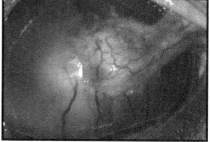

Figure 5-43 (left) Small and deep melting ulcer. Limbal vascularization is very active. The corneal edema prevents a view of the pupil.
Figure 5-44 (right) A conjunctival pedicle flap covers the ulcer in Figure 5-43 one week later.

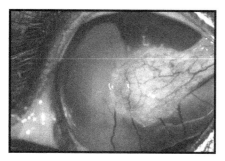
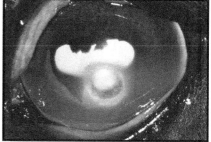

Figure 5-45 (left) The conjunctival flap is in place, and the cornea clearing of edema one week after photograph Figure 5-44.
Figure 5-46 (right) A melting ulcer has progressed to the formation of a thin "gutter" that nearly exposes Descemet's membrane.

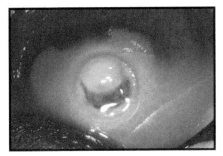
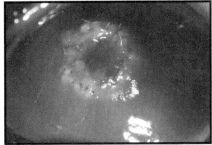

Figure 5-47 (left) More edema is present adjacent to the dark "gutter" one day later in the eye in Figure 5-46.

Figure 5-48 (right) A corneal transplant to remove and replace the necrotic tissue was performed. A conjunctival pedicle flap then covered the graft.

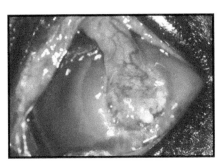
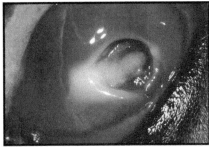

Figure 5-49 (left) Three weeks after the surgery in Figure 5-48 the cornea is healing with a large scar.

Figure 5-50 (right) A deep melting ulcer with a posterior corneal, yellow-white layer is present.

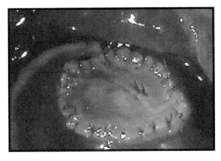
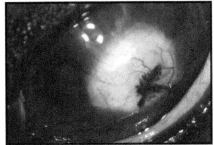

Figure 5-51 (left) A full thickness corneal transplant removes and replaces the necrotic tissue in the eye in Figure 5-50.

Figure 5-52 (right) A prominent scar covers the transplant site in Figure 5-50 three months postoperatively. The pupil remains miotic.

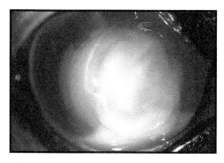
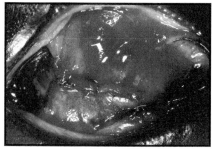

Figure 5-53 (left) A large diameter melting corneal ulcer caused by Pseudomonas has hypopyon.

Figure 5-54 (right) A conjunctival hood flap covers the ulcer site in the eye in Figure 5-53.

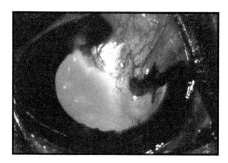
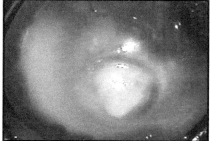

Figure 5-55 (left) The conjunctival graft remains partially in place, but uveitis is absent and the cornea clearing one month after placement in the eye in Figure 5-53.

Figure 5-56 (right) A melting fungal ulcer with severe corneal edema and uveitis.

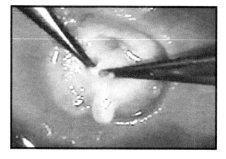
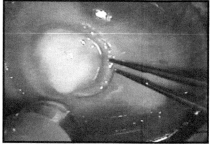

Figure 5-57 (left) Surgical removal of the necrotic cornea speeds healing.

Figure 5-58 (right) A biopsy punch is used to trephine the full thickness necrotic ulcer in the eye in Figure 5-56.

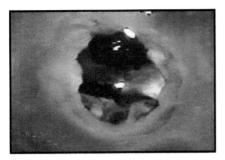
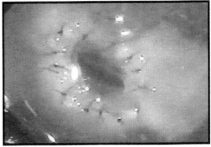

Figure 5-59 (left) Intraoperative photograph of the iris and tapetal reflection through the pupil are present after corneal removal in the eye in Figure 5-58.

Figure 5-60 (right) A full thickness corneal transplant graft is used for therapy in the eye in Figure 5-59.

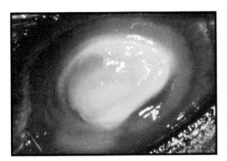
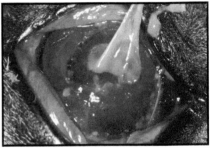

Figure 5-61 (left) Large Aspergillus and Pseudomonas melting ulcer in an Arab stallion. Note thin, ventral crescent shaped areas.

Figure 5-62 (right) Severe melting associated with the fungus *Acremonium* in a mare.

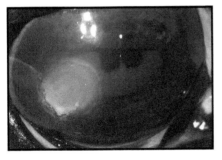
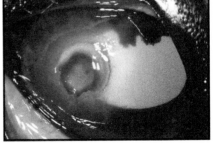

Figure 5-63 (left) Fluorescein dye is retained in a fungal ulcer.

Figure 5-64 (right) Two weeks later the eye in Figure 5-63 has developed a thick brown fungal plaque. A crescent shaped area of corneal thinning is found adjacent to the right of the plaque.

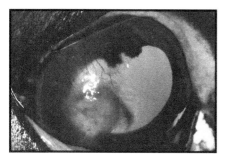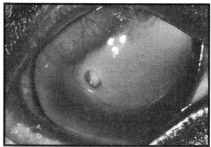

Figure 5-65 (left) The ulcer has resolved and healed 26 days since therapy began in the eye in Figure 5-63.

Figure 5-66 (right) A small descemetocele associated with a fungus is present.

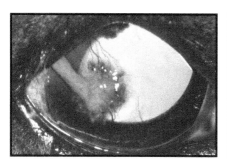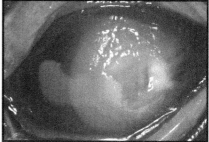

Figure 5-67 (left) A conjunctival graft was placed on the ulcer in the eye in Figure 5-66. It is now healed thirty days later.

Figure 5-68 (right) A superficial fungal ulcer with signs of melting is present. Medical therapy was instituted.

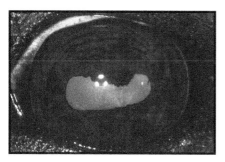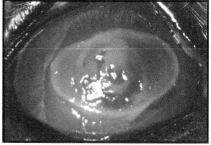

Figure 5-69 (left) This is the eye in Figure 5-68 five years later. Little scarring is present.

Figure 5-70 (right) A large brown fungal plaque is present with thin areas of cornea near the ventral ulcer margin.

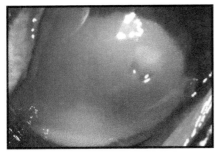
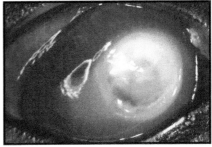

Figure 5-71 (left) A small yellow fungal ulcer with severe generalized corneal edema and hypopyon is present.

Figure 5-72 (right) A large and melting fungal ulcer has blood vessels approaching the dorsal ulcer edge. A conjunctival graft was placed.

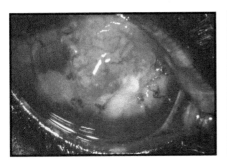
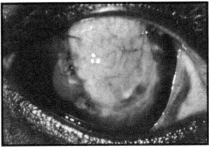

Figure 5-73 (left) The graft is partially dehisced in the eye in Figure 5-72 one week after surgery.

Figure 5-74 (right) The cornea is clearing and the uveitis absent 2.5 weeks after graft placement in the eye in Figure 5-72.

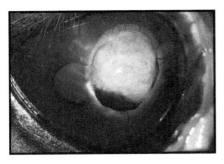
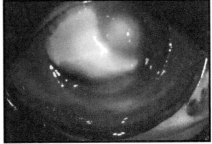

Figure 5-75 (left) A large scar remains from the conjunctival graft six weeks post-operatively in the eye in Figure 5-72. The scar is beginning to pigment ventrally.

Figure 5-76 (right) This melting ulcer is large and has a thin crescent shaped "gutter" or furrow ventrally.

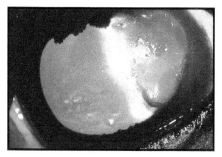 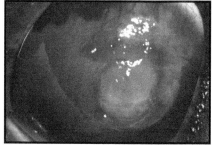

Figure 5-77 (left) Large melting fungal ulcer with lateral vascularization at the edge of the fungal plaque. The pupil is dilated from atropine.

Figure 5-78 (right) Three weeks later the eye in Figure 5-77 displays more vascularization but melting is still prominent.

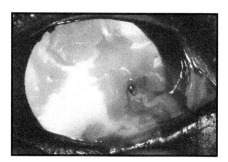 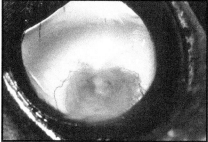

Figure 5-79 (left) A flow of aqueous humor leaking from a fistula or hole in the middle of an ulcer changes the color of fluorescein dye applied to the cornea. (Positive Seidel's Test; Video 22).

Figure 5-80 (right) Two weeks later the fistula in Figure 5-79 is still present and seen as a small dark spot in the center of a vascularizing fungal ulcer.

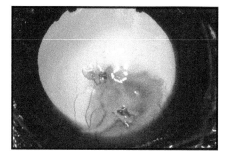 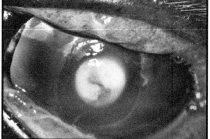

Figure 5-81 (left) The fistula was sutured and the fistula closed. The photo is two weeks after the image in Figure 5-80.

Figure 5-82 (right) A melting ulcer caused by *Staphylococcus*.

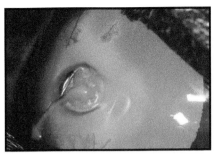
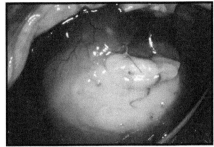

Figure 5-83 (left) A melting ulcer with a descemetocele was treated with a conjunctival flap.

Figure 5-84 (right) The conjunctival flap in the eye in figure 5-83 was trimmed six weeks postoperatively.

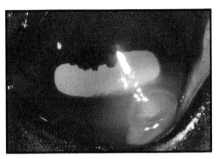
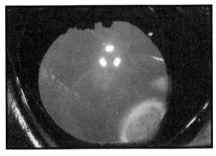

Figure 5-85 (left) A focal melting ulcer and slight corneal edema in a foal.

Figure 5-86 (right) The ulcer in Figure 5-85 is healed after six weeks of medical therapy.

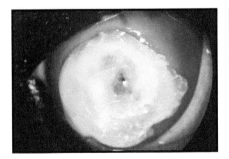
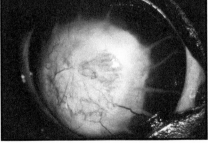

Figure 5-87 (left) A small central descemetocele (dark spot) is present in this melting ulcer caused by *Staphylococcus*. It was treated with a total conjunctival flap.

Figure 5-88 (right) The cornea is scarred in the eye in Figure 5-87 one month after conjunctival flap placement. The horse has limited vision. Large conjunctival flaps leave large scars.

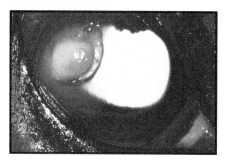
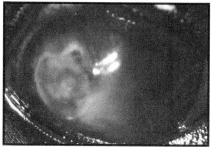

Figure 5-89 (left) Deep crescent shaped ulcer is nasal to a melting ulcer.

Figure 5-90 (right) Two weeks of medical therapy result in granulation tissue in the eye in Figure 5-89.

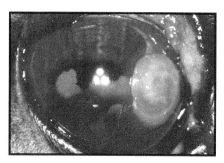
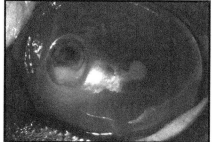

Figure 5-91 (left) Hyphema from a torn corpora nigra is found in an eye with a melting corneal ulcer.

Figure 5-92 (right) Deep melting ulcer and miotic pupil from uveitis in an eye with Streptococcus infection.

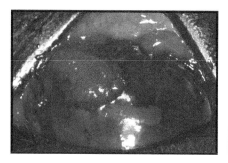
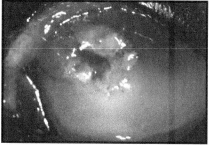

Figure 5-93 (left) A conjunctival pedicle flap is placed over the ulcer in Figure 5-92.

Figure 5-94 (right) Two days after the flap placement in the eye in Figure 5-92, the flap is being digested by tear film proteinases. Hypopyon is present.

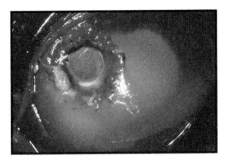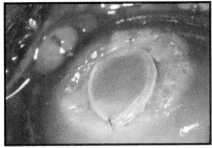

Figure 5-95 (left) Four days after the image in Figure 5-94, a descemetocele is present following surgical removal of the flap.

Figure 5-96 (right) A corneal transplant is performed on the eye in Figure 5-95.

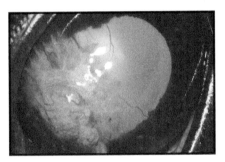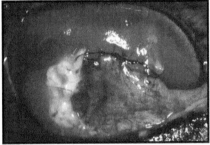

Figure 5-97 (left) The transplant is healed by scarring one month after the Figure 5-95 photo.

Figure 5-98 (right) Streptococcus abscesses and a descemetocele are present. The conjunctival flap is retracting to expose the deep ulcer.

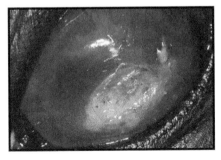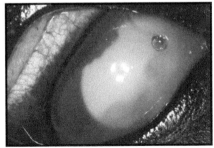

Figure 5-99 (left) A large diameter central ulcer due to tear dessication from inability to blink in facial nerve paralysis.

Figure 5-100 (right) A small descemetocele, corneal edema, and fibrin in the anterior chamber are found in this horse. A conjunctival flap was placed.

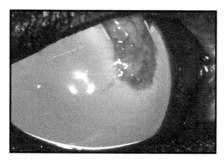
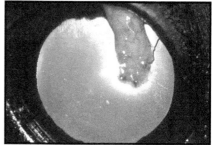

Figure 5-101 (left) The flap in Figure 5-100 two weeks postoperatively.
Figure 5-102 (right) The flap in Figure 5-100 four weeks postoperatively.

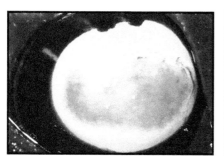
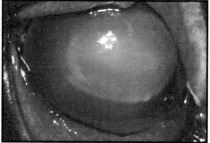

Figure 5-103 (left) A superficial Aspergillus fungal ulcer is present.
Figure 5-104 (right) The fungal plaque is more prominent 3 days after the image in Figure 5-103.

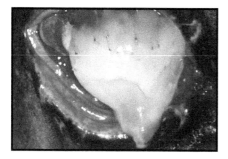
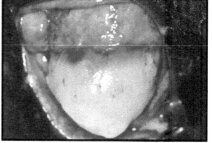

Figure 5-105 (left) Severe melting from Pseudomonas and Aspergillus is present 28 days after the image in Figure 5-103.
Figure 5-106 (right) Amniotic membrane covers the entire cornea but sloughed off and was covered with a conjunctival flap.

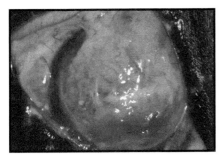 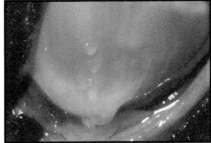

Figure 5-107 (left) Vascularization is present six weeks after the image in Figure 5-103. Severe scarring limits vision due to the conjunctival flap.

Figure 5-108 (right) Deep melting ulcer involving the entire cornea due to fungus and bacteria. This is an example of the "catastrophic" cornea. A double amnion graft was placed.

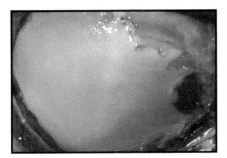 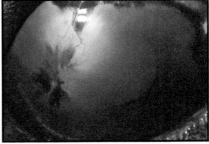

Figure 5-109 (left) Ten days postoperatively the amnion is intact.

Figure 5-110 (right) Four months after surgery the eye in Figure 5-108 has little corneal scarring and is visual. The pigmented area is where the amnion was incorporated into the cornea. The clear area is where the amnion was not retained.

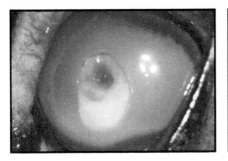 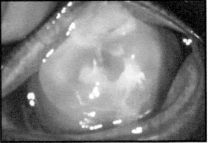

Figure 5-111 (left) Melting ulcer with white necrotic center, corneal edema, peripheral vascularization, and hypopyon.

Figure 5-112 (right) *Shewanella* infection causes massive melting.

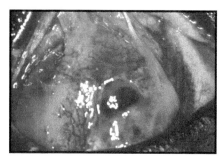
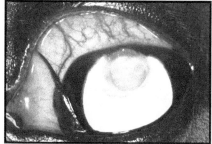

Figure 5-113 (left) Iris prolapse following conjunctival flap placement in the eye in Figure 5-112.

Figure 5-114 (right) Melting ulcer in dorsal cornea treated with conjunctival flap.

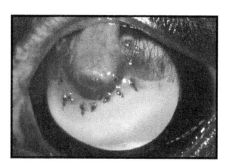
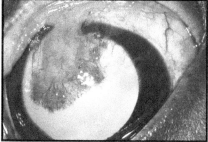

Figure 5-115 (left) Eye in Figure 5-113 12 days postoperatively. Vascularization surrounds the graft.

Figure 5-116 (right) Eye in Figure 5-113 21 days postoperatively.

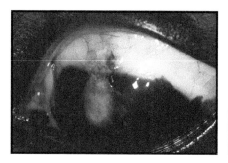
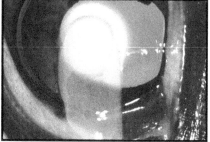

Figure 5-117 (left) Eye in Figure 5-113 55 days postoperatively. The flap has been trimmed.

Figure 5-118 (right) Cornea is so liquefied that it is "running" down the cornea in this melting ulcer.

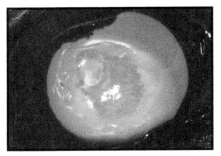 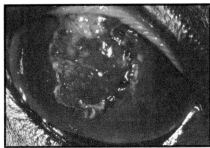

Figure 5-119 (left) Large diameter fungal ulcer is treated with a conjunctival flap.
Figure 5-120 (right) Conjunctival flap from the eye in Figure 5-119 one day post-operatively.

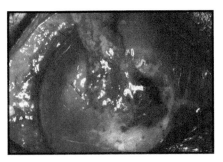 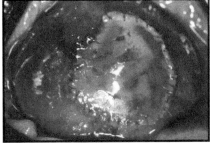

Figure 5-121 (left) The flap is retracting and an iris prolapse present five days after flap placement.
Figure 5-122 (right) An amniotic membrane covers the iris prolapse prior to conjunctival flap surgery in the eye in Figure 5-121.

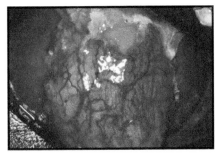 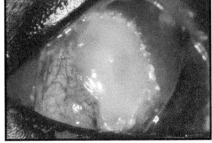

Figure 5-123 (left) Five days following the second surgery the conjunctival flap is retracting slightly in the eye in Figure 5-119.
Figure 5-124 (right) The flap in Figure 5-123 has retracted three days later to show the amniotic membrane still in place.

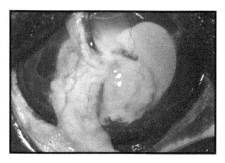
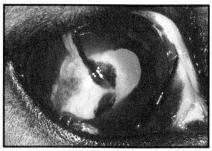

Figure 5-125 (left) A third conjunctival flap is in place 35 days after the image in Figure 5-123.

Figure 5-126 (right) The conjunctival flap is pigmenting 70 days after the image in Figure 5-125. The eye is visual.

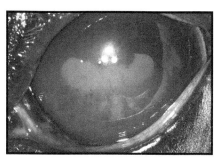
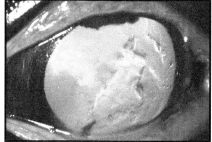

Figure 5-127 (left) Slight rose bengal retention and corneal edema are present in this horse with very early keratomycosis and glaucoma.

Figure 5-128 (right) A superficial fungal ulcer is lightly fluorescein positive with rose bengal retention at the edges of the ulcer.

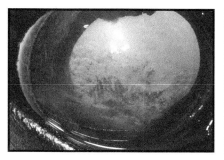
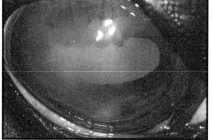

Figure 5-129 (left) Two years later the horse in Figure 5-128 is mildly painful, fluorescein negative, and rose bengal positive. Aspergillus was cultured from the rose bengal site.

Figure 5-130 (right) One month later, the horse in Figure 5-129 has some corneal edema and slight peripheral vascularization following antifungal drug administration.

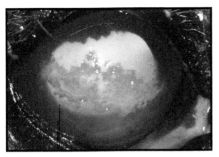
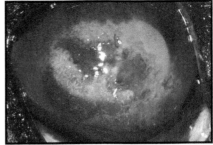

Figure 5-131 (left) Fungal plaques are partially fluorescein positive in this horse.

Figure 5-132 (right) Rose bengal retention is prominent over the fungi in the horse in Figure 5-131.

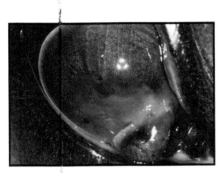
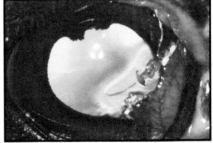

Figure 5-133 (left) An iris prolapse caused by a corneal laceration is present ventro-nasally. The pupil is miotic and obsctructed by fibrin.

Figure 5-134 (right) Five days postoperatively, the horse in Figure 5-133 has a dilated pupil and anterior chamber restoration following suturing of the corneal laceration and conjunctival flap placement.

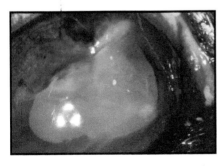
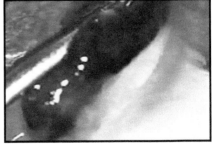

Figure 5-135 (left) An iris prolapse dorsally due to a laceration. Fibrin is present in the anterior chamber.

Figure 5-136 (right) An attempt is made to push the iris back into the anterior chamber in the eye in Figure 5-135 prior to suturing the cornea.

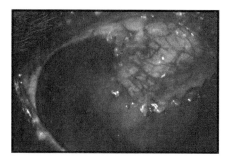 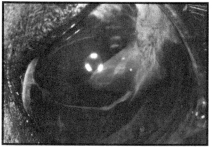

Figure 5-137 (left) Five days postoperatively, the pupil is slightly dilated and the cornea cloudy following corneal suturing and conjunctival flap surgery in the eye in Figure 5-136.

Figure 5-138 (right) Severe scarring, a relatively small pupil and early cataract formation are present 4 months postoperatively in the horse in Figure 5-136.

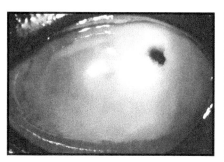 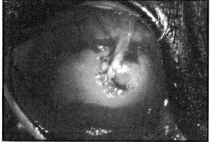

Figure 5-139 (left) An iris prolapse due to a melting ulcer with heavy fibrin deposition in the anterior chamber is treated by corneal transplantation and a conjunctival graft.

Figure 5-140 (right) Twelve days later, the horse in Figure 5-139 has the conjunctival flap retracting and exposing the corneal transplant.

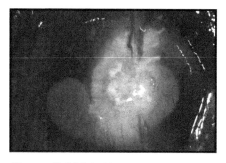 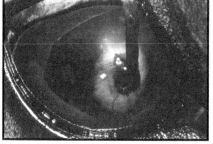

Figure 5-141 (left) One month postoperatively, the horse in Figure 5-139 has some corneal scarring but is visual with no uveitis.

Figure 5-142 (right) One year postoperatively, the horse in Figure 5-139 has corneal scarring and pigmentation of the conjunctival graft.

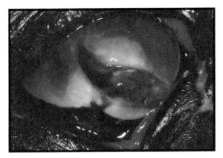 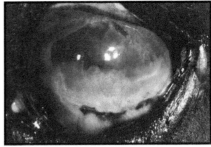

Figure 5-143 (left) Very large iris prolapse. No dazzle reflex was present but the owner declined enucleation.

Figure 5-144 (right) A large corneal scar is present one month postoperatively in the horse in Figure 5-143. The eye is blind and nonpainful.

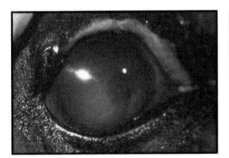 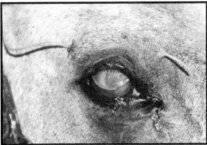

Figure 5-145 (left) A central air bubble is between the contact lens and the cornea in a horse treated for a superficial corneal ulcer.

Figure 5-146 (right) The subpalpebral lavage tubing is loose and causing corneal ulceration in this horse.

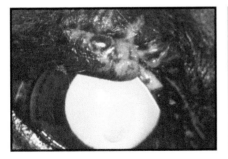 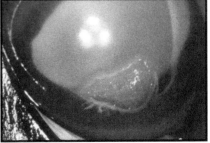

Figure 5-147 (left) Scarring from a lid laceration resulted in a superficial ulcer.

Figure 5-148 (right) A superficial noninfected corneal ulcer has occurred following surgical vitrectomy.

Proteinases in the Tear Film

✓ Tear film proteinases normally provide a surveillance and repair function to detect and remove damaged cells or collagen caused by regular wear and tear of the cornea. These enzymes exist in a balance with inhibitory factors to prevent excessive degradation of normal tissue.

✓ Two major families of proteinases that may affect the cornea include the matrix metalloproteinases (MMP) and the serine proteinase neutrophil elastase (NE). MMPs appear to predominate in the direct breakdown of stromal collagen in the horse. Tear MMP-2 levels are increased by 83%, and MMP-9 levels increased by 232% in eyes with ulcers. The tear NE levels are two to four times normal but do not directly cause collagenase activity. They presumedly induce degenerative corneal change by upregulating other tear and corneal factors that promote corneal degeneration.

♥ Bacterial and fungal pathogens induce corneal epithelial cells, corneal stromal fibroblasts, and leukocytes (PMN) in the tear film to upregulate cytokines (see Figures 1-9, 2-7, 2-12, 5-5, 5-23, 5-24), and (Figure 5-149) that induce MMP production and elicit inflammatory and degradative processes.

✓ Proteinases that may contribute to corneal ulceration in the early stages of infection could be of bacterial or corneal cell origin. In the later stages as PMNs accumulate, PMN-derived proteinases predominate as the main factor in corneal tissue destruction. Tear film MMP-2, MMP-9 and NE are elevated in the eyes of horses with ulcers.

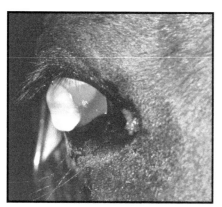

Figure 5-149 White gelatinous tissue indicative of corneal "melting".

✓ In pathologic processes such as ulcerative keratitis, excessive levels of these proteinases can lead to rapid degeneration of collagen and other components of the stroma, potentially inducing keratomalacia or corneal "melting" (see Figures 5-6, 5-14, 5-17, 5-23 to 5-25, 5-28, 5-29, 5-43 to 5-60, 5-62, 5-76, 5-77, 5-82 to 5-97, 5-99, 5-100, 5-108 to 5-126, 5-149) and (Figures 5-150 and 5-151).

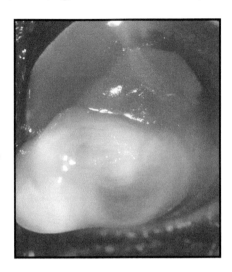

Figure 5-150 Close-up of the eye in Figure 5-149 demonstrates the severe degree of corneal collagen breakdown.

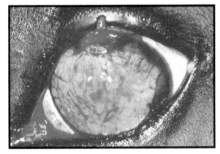

Figure 5-151 A large conjunctival flap resulted in globe survival but limited vision due to severe corneal scarring 6 weeks postoperatively in the horse from Figures 5-149 and 5-150.

Corneal Sensitivity in Foals and Adult Horses

✓ Corneal sensation is important for corneal healing. The cornea of the adult horse is very sensitive compared to other animals such as the dog and cat.

✓ Corneal touch threshold analysis revealed the corneas of sick or hospitalized foals were significantly less sensitive than those of adult horses or normal foals. The incidence of corneal disease is also much higher in sick neonates than in healthy foals of similar age. (Figure 5-153) Corneal sensation can be reduced in horses with EPM.

⚷ Ulcerative keratitis in the equine neonate often differs from adult horses in clinical signs and disease course. Foals may not show characteristic epiphora, blepharospasm, or conjunctivitis, and the ulcers may be missed without daily fluorescein staining. This decreased sensitivity may partially explain the lack of clinical signs often seen in sick neonates with corneal ulcers.

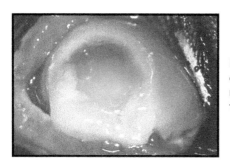

Figure 5-152 A large thin area of cornea caused by severe corneal stromal melting. Total corneal melting is termed the "catastophic cornea."

Corneal Healing in the Horse

⚷ The thickness of the equine cornea is 1.0 to 1.5 mm in the center and 0.8 mm at the periphery.

⚷ The normal equine corneal epithelium is 8 to 10 cell layers thick, but increases to 10 to 15 cell layers thick with hypertrophy of the basal epithelial cells following corneal injury. The epithelial basement membrane is not completely formed six weeks following corneal injury in the horse, in spite of the epithelium completely covering the ulcer site.

♥ Healing of large diameter, superficial, noninfected corneal ulcers is generally rapid and linear for 5-7 days, and then slows. Healing of ulcers in the second eye may be slower than in the first and is related to increased tear proteinase activity. Healing time of a 7-mm diameter, midstromal depth, noninfected corneal trephine wound was nearly 12 days in horses (0.6 mm/day).

✓ The cornea vascularizes at about 1 mm/day.

✓ Neutrophils move into the corneal stroma at about 8.6 mm/day.

✓ Horse corneas demonstrate a pronounced fibrovascular healing response. The unique corneal healing properties of the horse in regards to excessive corneal vascularization and fibrosis appear to be strongly species specific (see Figures 5-18, 5-30, 5-65, 5-67, 5-75,

5-84, 5-86, 5-88, 5-90, 5-97, 5-102, 5-126, 5-141, 5-144, 5-146) and (Figure 5-153).

🗝 Lack of ulcer progression equals improvement in infectious keratitis. Corneal healing does not occur till the tear film and stromal proteinase activity is reduced. The corneal destruction must be stabilized before it can heal. Treatments must reduce tear MMP levels by up to 80% before ulcer healing can occur.

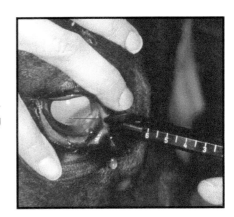

Figure 5-153 Corneal sensation is measured with a Cochet-Bonnet aesthesiometer in a horse with a small melting corneal ulcer.

The Equine Corneal Microenvironment

The environment of the horse is such that the conjunctiva and cornea are constantly exposed to bacteria and fungi.

✓ The corneal epithelium of the horse is a formidable barrier to the colonization and invasion of potentially pathogenic bacteria or fungi normally present on the surface of the horse cornea and conjunctiva.

✓ A defect in the corneal epithelium allows bacteria or fungi to adhere to the cornea and to initiate infection. *Staphylococcus, Streptococcus, Pseudomonas, Aspergillus,* and *Fusarium* spp. are common causes of corneal ulceration in the horse (see Figures 5-24, 5-25) and (Figure 5-154).

🗝 Infection should be considered likely in every corneal ulcer in the horse but should not be the only consideration in the progression of an ulcer. Fungal involvement should be suspected if there is a history of corneal injury with vegetative material, or if a corneal ulcer has received prolonged antibiotic and/or corticosteroid therapy with slight or no improvement.

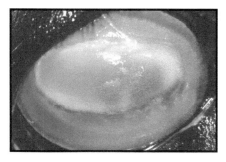

Figure 5-154 Large yellow-brown fungal plaque covers most of the cornea in this horse.

♥ Tear film neutrophils and some bacteria and fungi are associated with highly destructive proteinase and collagenase enzymes that can result in rapid corneal stromal thinning, descemetocele formation, and perforation. Excessive proteinase activity is termed "melting", and results in a liquified, grayish-gelatinous appearance to the stroma near the margin of the ulcer (see Figures 5-25, 5-32, 5-33, 5-43, 5-47, 5-50, 5-53, 5-56, 5-83, 5-87, 5-89, 5-105, 5-108, 5-112, 5-118, 5-119 5-149, 5-150, 5-151, and 5-154). It is important to break the molecular momentum of these proteases in treating infected and sterile ulcers.

♥ Total corneal ulceration ultimately requires the degradation of collagen that forms the framework of the corneal stroma. Melting of the entire cornea is potentially "catastrophic" for the eye.

☛ Many early cases of equine ulcerative keratitis present, initially, as minor corneal epithelial ulcers or infiltrates, with slight pain, blepharospasm, epiphora and photophobia. At first anterior uveitis and corneal vascularization may not be clinically pronounced. Slight droopiness of the eyelashes of the upper eyelid may be an early, yet subtle sign of corneal ulceration.

✋ A vicious cycle may be initiated after the first injury to the cornea, with "second injury to the cornea" occurring because of the action of inflammatory cytokines.

☛ Ulcers, uveitis, blepharitis, conjunctivitis, glaucoma, and dacryocystitis must be considered in the differential for the horse with a painful eye.

✓ Corneal edema may surround the ulcer or involve the entire cornea.

☛ Signs of anterior uveitis are found with every corneal ulcer in the horse, and include miosis, fibrin, hyphema or hypopyon (see Figures 5-6, 5-7, 5-11, 5-20, 5-21, 5-26, 5-53, 5-56, 5-71, 5-91, 5-94, 5-133).

✓ Persistent superficial ulcers may become indolent due to hyaline membrane formation on the ulcer bed.

❀ Fluorescein dye retention is diagnostic of a full thickness epithelial defect or corneal ulcer. Faint fluorescein retention may indicate a microerosion or partial epithelial cell layer defect due to infiltration of fluorescein dye between inflamed epithelial cell junctions.

♥ All corneal injuries should be fluorescein stained to detect corneal ulcers. Fluorescein should be used at full strength and not be diluted or false negative results can occur.

� Rose bengal retention indicates a defect in or instability of the mucin layer of the tear film (see Figures 5-129, 5-130, 5-132, and 4-54). It will also stain the corneal stroma if the mucin layer is absent. An ulcer that stains positive for fluorescein and rose Bengal may have a worse prognosis as the tear film is unstable.

❀ Horses with painful eyes need to have their corneas stained with both fluorescein dye and rose bengal dye as fungal ulcers in the earliest stage will be negative to the fluorescein but positive for the rose bengal.

✋ Fungi may induce changes in the tear film mucin layer prior to attachment to the cornea. Early fungal lesions that retain rose bengal are multifocal in appearance and may be mistaken for viral keratitis.

� Microbiologic culture and sensitivity for bacteria and fungi are recommended for horses with rapidly progressive, and deep corneal ulcers. Corneal cultures should be obtained first and then followed by corneal scrapings for cytology. Mixed bacterial and fungal infections can be present.

✓ Vigorous corneal scraping at the edge and base of a corneal ulcer is used to detect bacteria and fungal hyphae. Samples can be obtained with the handle end of a sterile scalpel blade and topical anesthesia. Superficial scraping with a cotton swab cannot be expected to yield organisms in a high percentage of cases.

♥ A "crater-like" defect that retains fluorescein dye at its periphery and is clear in the center is a descemetocele, and indicates the globe is at high risk of rupture. Descemet's membrane does not retain fluorescein dye, whereas deep ulcers that continue to have stroma anterior to Descemet's membrane will retain fluorescein (see Figures 5-9 and 5-10)

♥ Deep penetration of the stroma to Descemet's membrane with perforation of the cornea is a possible sequelae to all corneal ulcers in horses.

Medical Therapy

♥ Once a corneal ulcer is diagnosed, the therapy must be carefully considered to ensure comprehensive treatment. Medical therapy almost always comprises the initial major thrust in ulcer control, albeit tempered by judicious use of adjunctive surgical procedures. This intensive pharmacological attack should be modified according to its efficacy.

✓ ⊙ Subpalpebral or nasolacrimal lavage treatment systems are employed to treat a fractious horse or one with a painful eye that needs frequent therapy (Figure 5-155) (Video 6).

☋⊸ The clarity of the cornea, the depth and size of the ulcer, the degree of corneal vascularization, the amount of tearing, the pupil size, and intensity of the anterior uveitis should be monitored. Serial fluorescein staining of the ulcer is indicated to assess healing.

☋⊸ As the cornea heals the stimulus for the uveitis will diminish, and the pupil will dilate with minimal atropine therapy.

✓ Self-trauma should be reduced with hard or soft cup hoods.

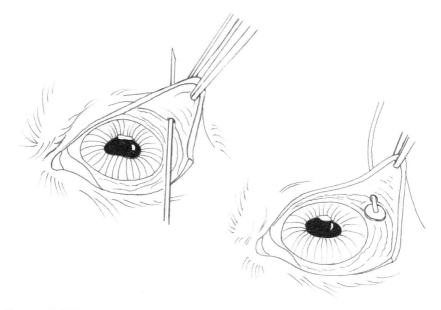

Figure 5-155 Installation of subpalpebral lavage system for topical medical treatment is often a necessity in horses. One-hole systems with a footplate in the conjunctival fornix of the upper or lower eyelid are preferred.

Antibiotics

🔑 Bacterial and fungal growth must be halted and the microbes rendered non-viable. Broad- spectrum topical antibiotics are usually administered with culture and sensitivity tests aiding selection. Topical antibiotic solutions interfere with corneal epithelial healing less than ointments. Gentamicin should be used in ulcers with evidence of stromal melting only.

♥ Topically applied antibiotics, such as chloramphenicol, gramicidin-neomycin-polymyxin B, gentamicin, ciprofloxacin, 1% doxycycline or tobramycin ophthalmic solutions may be utilized to treat bacterial ulcers. Frequency of medication varies from q2h to q8h.

♥ Cefazolin (55mg/ml), chloramphenicol, bacitracin, and carbenicillin are effective against beta hemolytic Streptococcus.

♥ Ciprofloxacin, amikacin (10 mg/ml), and polymyxin B (0.25% IV solution) may be used topically for gentamicin resistant Pseudomonas.

Collagenolysis Prevention

Activation and/or production of proteolytic enzymes by corneal epithelial cells, leucocytes and microbial organisms are responsible for stromal collagenolysis or "melting".

✋ Severe corneal inflammation secondary to bacterial (especially, Pseudomonas and beta hemolytic Streptococcus) or fungal infection may result in sudden, rapid corneal liquefaction and perforation. Excessive proteinase activity can also occur in sterile ulcers!

✋ Autogenous serum administered topically can reduce tear film and corneal protease activity in corneal ulcers in horses. Serum is biologically nontoxic and contains an alpha-2 macroglobulin with antiproteinase activity.

🔑 The serum can be administered topically as often as possible, and should be replaced by new serum every 5-8 days.

✓ Five to 10% acetylcysteine, and/or 0.17% sodium EDTA can be instilled hourly, in addition to the other indicated drugs, for antimelting effect until stromal liquefaction ceases.

✓ It may be necessary to use serum, EDTA, and acetylcysteine simultaneously in severe cases.

✓ Subconjunctival tetanus antitoxin contains macroglobulins with anticollagenase effects and can also slow corneal melting.

Treat Uveitis

☛ The uveitis associated with corneal ulcers can be mild to quite severe in the anterior part of the eye but is generally minimal, no matter how severe the anterior uveitis, in the posterior segment. The uveitis must be treated medically.

☛ Atropine sulfate is a common therapeutic agent for equine eye problems. Topically applied atropine (1%) is effective in stabilizing the blood-aqueous barrier, reducing vascular protein leakage, minimizing pain from ciliary muscle spasm, and reducing the chance of synechia formation by causing pupillary dilatation.

☛ Atropine may be utilized topically q4h to q6h with the frequency of administration reduced as soon as the pupil dilates. 2.5% phenylephrine can be used with atropine to achieve mydriasis.

☛ Miosis can be difficult to overcome as synechia can rapidly occur in minutes following fibrin formation in the anterior chamber.

💣 Topical atropine has been shown to prolong intestinal transit time, reduce and abolish intestinal sounds, and diminish the normal myoelectric patterns in the small intestine and large colon of horses. Some horses appear more sensitive than others to these atropine effects, and may "respond" by displaying signs of colic and/or prolonged intestinal transit time.

💣 Cecal impaction may occur secondary to topical atropine administration.

♥ Horses receiving topically administered atropine should be monitored for signs of colic, even though a single 50 microliter drop of 1% atropine only contains 0.5 mg of the drug!

☛ Systemically administered NSAIDs such as phenylbutazone (1 gm BID PO) or flunixin meglumine (1 mg/kg BID, IV, IM or PO) can be used orally or parenterally, and are effective in reducing uveal exudation and relieving ocular discomfort from the anterior uveitis in horses with ulcers.

☛ Topical nonsteroidal antiinflammatory drugs (NSAIDs) such as profenol, flurpbiprofen and diclofenamic acid (BID to TID) can also reduce the degree of uveitis.

♥ Horses with corneal ulcers and secondary uveitis should be stall-rested till the condition is healed. Intraocular hemorrhage and increased severity of uveitis are sequelae to overexertion.

Adjunctive Surgical Therapy

Bandage Soft Contact Lens (SCL)

✓ Bandage SCLs help to maintain apposition of the healing epithelium to the stroma, reduce pain, and protect the new epithelium. Disadvantages include an occasional poor fit in horses thereby resulting in limited retention times. Contact lens retention time may be improved by partial temporary lateral tarsorrhaphy (see Figure 5-145).

Debridement, Keratectomy and Keratotomy

⊗⊸ Removing necrotic tissue and microbial debris by keratectomy speeds healing, minimizes scarring, and decreases the stimulus for iridocyclitis.

⊗⊸ Persistent superficial ulcers may need surgical debridement and keratotomy to remove the hyaline membrane slowing epithelial healing.

✓ Debridement to remove abnormal epithelium of refractory superficial erosions can be accomplished with topical anesthesia and a cotton-tipped applicator.

✓ Superficial punctate or grid keratotomy of superficial ulcers with a 20-gauge needle can increase the ability of the epithelial cells to migrate and adhere to the ulcer surface (see Figures 5-3, 5-4, 5-36) and (Figure 5-156).

💣 Punctate and grid keratotomies are only used for superficial, noninfectious ulcers or infection can result (see Figures 5-5, 5-32 and 5-33).

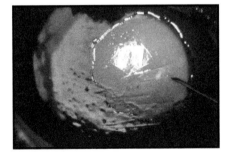

Figure 5-156 A grid keratotomy with a 20 gauge needle is used to treat a superficial noninfected ulcer.

Conjunctival Flaps

✓ ⊙ Conjunctival grafts or flaps are used frequently in equine ophthalmology for the clinical management of deep, melting, and large corneal ulcers, descemetoceles, and for perforated corneal ulcers with and without iris prolapse (Figures 5-157, 5-158, and 5-159) (Video 1).

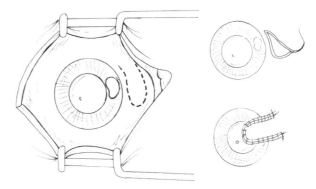

Figure 5-157 Pedicle conjunctival grafts are used for ulcers 2 to 12 mm in diameter (left). The conjunctiva adjacent to the ulcer is undermined (upper right) and rotated to cover the ulcer such that little tension is present in the graft to cause graft retraction. Sutures placed into the cornea and the conjunctival graft hold it in place such that the graft adheres to the ulcer site (lower right).

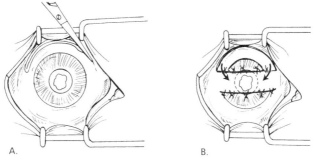

A.   B.

Figure 5-158 Bipedicle conjunctival grafts are used for melting ulcers, large ulcers, and to replace pedicle flaps that have retracted from the ulcer site. The conjunctival graft remains attached at two sites and the graft is sutured to the cornea.

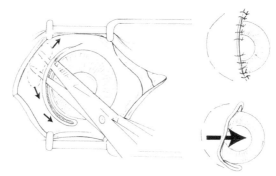

Figure 5-159 Hood conjunctival flaps are used to cover ulcers involving the majority of the cornea. Severe corneal scarring usually results. The conjunctiva is mobilized at the limbus (left), undermined towards the fornix, and pulled towards the corneal ulcer (lower right). It is then sutured to the cornea (upper right).

♥ To augment lost corneal thickness and strength, deep corneal ulcers threatening perforation may require conjunctival flap placement. Conjunctival flaps are associated with some scarring of the ulcer site (see Figures 5-7, 5-8, 5-11, 5-12, 5-17, 5-18, 5-20, 5-21, 5-22, 5-26, 5-27, 5-32, 5-33, 5-43 to 5-45, 5-49, 5-54, 5-67, 5-73, 5-75, 5-98, 5-101, 5-107, 5-109, 5-113, 5-115, 5-116, 5-117, 5-120 to 5-126, 5-137, 5-140, 5-141) and (Figures 5-160 to 5-164). Coverage with a 360°, hood, island, pedicle, or bridge flap should be maintained for 4 to 12 weeks. Necrosis of blood vessels in the flap can result in avascularity and poor function of the flap. Fungi can colonize the flap tissue. Leakage of aqueous humor under a flap can cause graft thickening and premature graft release. Tear film proteases will attack absorbable sutures attached to the conjunctival flap. Reoccurrence of the inflammation may occur following flap transection. Corneal transplants may be used in conjunction with conjunctival flaps (see Figures 5-48, 5-51, 5-60, and 5-96).

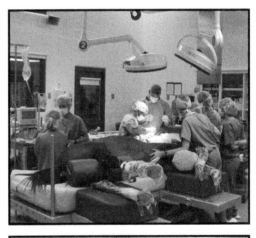

Figure 5-160 General anesthesia is used for this ophthalmic surgery in a horse.

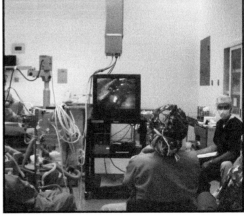

Figure 5-161 Students and visitors observe ophthalmic surgery on a video monitor at the University of Florida College of Veterinary Medicine in Gainesville, Florida, USA.

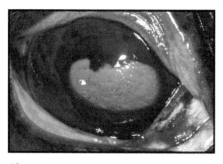
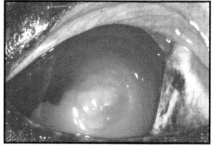

Figure 5-162 (left) Aspergillus causes disruption of the tear film and rose bengal dye retention prior to development of a fluorescein positive ulcer.

Figure 5-163 (right) Several weeks later a melting fungal ulcer has developed in the horse in Figure 5-162.

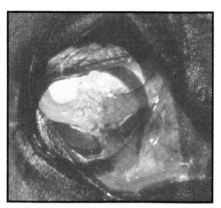

Figure 5-164 A conjunctival bipedicle graft is used to cover a large central corneal ulcer.

⚷ ⊙ A conjunctival pedicle flap is made by incising conjunctiva (excluding Tenon's capsule) 1-2 mm posterior to and parallel to the limbus with Steven's tenotomy scissors. The flap is undermined posteriorly toward the fornix as needed. A perpendicular incision is made at the distal end of the flap, and an incision parallel to the first incision and limbus is made several millimeters posterior to the first incision. The flap is rotated over the defect and sutured in place with absorbable 5-0 to 7-0 suture (see Figure 5-157) and (Figure 5-165) (Video 1).

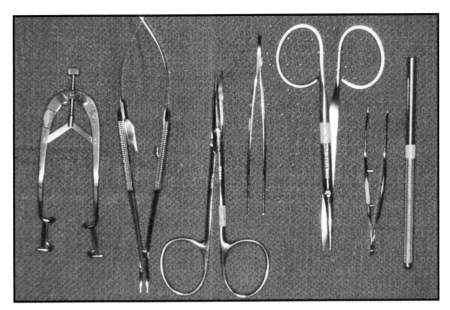

Figure 5-165 Surgical instruments necessary to perform basic ophthalmic surgical procedures include (left to right) eyelid speculum, microneedle holders, Steven's tenotomy scissors, Bishop Harmon forceps, small scissors, colibri forceps with 0.12 mm teeth, and a Beaver blade handle.

Amniotic Membrane Transplants

The amniotic membrane consists of an epithelium and stroma. It is a very strong yet thin tissue that is filled with antiproteinases and antiangiogenic substances. Amniotic membrane transplantation (AMT) may provide decreased fibrosis, reduced vascularization of corneal ulcers, and faster reepithelialization in horses with superficial and/or deep melting corneal ulcers. They most importantly act as a sink to remove proteinases and microbes, and attract neutrophils from the tears to reduce corneal liquefaction or melting. They may be used alone, or superficial or deep to conjunctival flaps. Single or multiple layers of AM can be used in deep or progressive melting ulcers, descemetoceles, and iris prolapses. AM placed over PK sites can reduce vascularization to preserve some graft transparency (see Figures 5-106, 5-122, 5-124) (Video 16).

Amniotic membrane transplants are highly recommended in catastrophic melting ulcers involving the entire cornea, and postkeratectomy for SCC. The scarring is dramatically less than with a conjunctival graft.

The AMT is stored epithelial side up on nitrocellulose paper in Dulbecco's Modified Eagle Medium with glycerol, penicillin, streptomycin, neomycin and amphotericin at -80C. The AM is allowed to thaw and washed with sterile saline (to wash off the glycerol) for 30 minutes. The stromal side is generally placed against the ulcer surface. The AM is sutured over the corneal lesion, or may be sutured at the limbus to cover the entire cornea. The AMT may be incorporated into the cornea or slough. I have found that if the AMT sloughs 7-10 days postoperaively that the corneal scarring is diminished compared to if the amnion is incorporated into the cornea.

Third-Eyelid (TE) Flap

✓ Nictitating membrane flaps are used for superficial corneal diseases including corneal erosions, neuroparalytic and neurotropic keratitis, temporary exposure keratitis, superficial corneal ulcers, superficial stromal abscesses, and to reinforce a bulbar conjunctival graft.

⚿ Formation of a third-eyelid flap with attachment to the upper eyelid is performed by placing 2-4 horizontal mattress sutures (Figure 5-166). Initially pass the cutting needle through the upper eyelid through the fornix at the desired location. Direct the needle (3-0 suture) through the anterior face of the TE approximately 3 mm from the leading edge, and then again in the skin through the fornix adjacent to the first bite. These sutures should not be full-thickness in the TE. One to three additional sutures are placed and then tied.

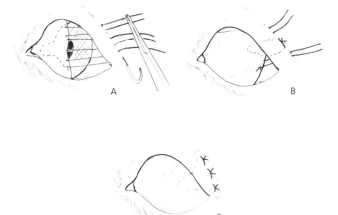

Figure 5-166 Third eyelid (TE) flap surgery involves placement of sutures in a horizontal direction through the lid skin and palpebral conjunctiva, through the TE cartilage, and then back through the conjunctiva and skin (A). The TE is pulled into the fornix and the sutures tied (B and C). Several sutures are necessary.

Temporary Tarsorrhaphy

✓ Horizontal mattress sutures enter the eyelid two to three millimeters from the eyelid margin with the cutting needle emerging from the central aspect (Meibomian gland line) of the eyelid margin, and then reentering the apposing lid margin to exit in the skin. 4-0 silk or nylon is commonly used for this procedure.

Enucleation

✓ Panophthalmitis following perforation of an infected corneal stromal ulcer has a poor prognosis. Phthisis bulbi is likely to result after a chronically painful course. Affected horses can be febrile and manifest signs of septicemia. To spare the unfortunate animal this discomfort, enucleation is the humane alternative. Histopathologic examination of the globe is recommended.

Inappropriate Therapy and Ulcers

✓ Topical corticosteroids may encourage growth of bacterial and fungal opportunists by interfering with non-specific inflammatory reactions and cellular immunity.

✋ Corticosteroid therapy by all routes is contraindicated in the management of corneal infections. Even topical corticosteroid instillation, to reduce the size of a corneal scar, may be disastrous if organisms remain indolent in the corneal stroma.

Important Concepts

💣 Corneal ulcers are frequently not clearly visible even with proper examination lighting

💣 All red or painful eyes must be stained with fluorescein and rose bengal dyes

💣 A slowly progressive, indolent course often belies the seriousness of the ulcer

💣 Corneal ulcers in horses may rapidly progress to descemetoceles

💣 Sterility of the ulcer does not necessarily equate with rapid healing

💣 Infection may persist to repopulate the corneal surface despite therapy

💣 Topical corticosteroids are contraindicated when the cornea retains fluorescein stain

💣 Miosis caused by a corneal ulcer or stromal abscess may be very difficult to overcome.

💣 Local anesthetics should not be used in treatment of corneal ulcers as they retard epithelial healing.

Corneal Lacerations/Perforations

✓ Ocular trauma is the result of a redistribution of kinetic energy and can have a variety of clinical manifestations.

🔑 Sharp, penetrating injuries have the forces localized to the site of impact. Blunt injuries carry a worse prognosis than injury from sharp objects or missiles as blunt forces are transmitted throughout the eye.

✓ Trauma from whips, nails, buckets, light fixtures, vegetative material, and tree branches can result in corneal/scleral lacerations. Injury to the lens, iris, and retina can accompany blunt or sharp corneal/scleral trauma. Improper suture placement of a corneal lesion can result in a fistula (see Figures 5-133 to 5-138, 5-143, 5-144) and (Figure 5-167).

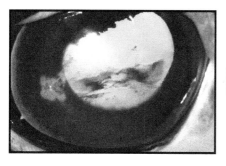

Figure 5-167 Small corneal laceration has caused hyphema in this horse eye.

🔑 Corneal lacerations in the horse are always accompanied by varying degrees of iridocyclitis. The eye may be cloudy, red, and painful. Blepharospasm and lacrimation are present with focal or generalized corneal edema. Slight droopiness of the eyelashes of the upper eyelid may be a subtle sign of corneal ulceration.

🔑 Full-thickness corneal/scleral perforations are usually associated with iris prolapse, shallow anterior chamber, and hyphema. If the corneal lesion extends to the limbus, the sclera should also be carefully checked for perforation because the scleral wound can be obscured by conjunctival chemosis and hemorrhage. Failure to detect a scleral tear will result in chronic hypotony and globe atrophy (phthisis bulbi).

✓ Ocular pain may also be found with corneal ulcers, uveitis, conjunctivitis, glaucoma, blepharitis, and dacryocystitis.

☞ Fluorescein dye staining of the cornea will reveal the laceration. Fluorescein dye may enter the anterior chamber. An ulcer that stains positive for fluorescein and rose Bengal may have a worse prognosis as the tear film is unstable.

☞ ⊙ The presence of a subtle, small corneal perforation or fistula is demonstrated by **Seidel's test** (see Figure 5-79) (Video 22). Streaming of clear aqueous humor into the fluorescein-stained tear film positively identifies the location of the leak. The concentration of fluorescein in the tear film must be very high. The horse's lids are held open, and a moistened fluorescein-impregnated paper strip applied over the area in question. When the test is positive, unstained aqueous humor is seen flowing through the more concentrated orange-red (green if viewed in cobalt-blue light) dye. As aqueous humor may leak intermittently from the wound when the intraocular pressure is extremely low, gentle pressure on the cornea with a cotton swab should be applied if a leak is not immediately apparent.

✓ Small corneal lacerations can heal quickly if surgical and medical therapy is prompt. Larger lesions are associated with more uveitis and will be slower to heal.

✓ Medical therapy is similar as for ulcers and should be sufficient for superficial, nonperforating lacerations. Topically applied antibiotics, atropine and serum, and systemic NSAIDs are recommended.

✓ Systemic NSAIDs and broad-spectrum parenteral antibiotics are also indicated for full thickness lesions.

✓ Deep or irregular corneal lacerations require surgical support of the cornea and more aggressive therapy for iridocyclitis and infection. Direct corneal suturing and conjunctival flaps are indicated to more rapidly restore corneal integrity.

☞ Both small and large full thickness corneal perforations should be surgically repaired. Complications include infection, iris prolapse, anterior synechiae, cataract formation, and persistent iridocyclitis. Both small and large corneal or scleral full thickness defects can result in phthisis bulbi if left untreated.

✓ A horse eye with a traumatic corneal perforation that has extensive extrusion of intraocular contents, severe intraocular hemorrhage, or evidence of bacterial infection should have the affected globe enucleated.

✓ Septic intrusion into the globe results in painful endophthalmitis. Such infection can spread to surrounding soft tissues and necessitates enucleation.

Fungal Ulcers in Horses

✓ Fungi are normal inhabitants of the equine environment and conjunctival microflora, but can become pathogenic following corneal injury.

✓ Aspergillus, Fusarium, Cylindrocarpon, Curvularia, Penicillium, Cystodendron, yeasts, and molds are known causes of fungal ulceration in horses.

☗ Ulcerative keratomycosis is a serious, sight-threatening disease in the horse. Blindness can occur (see Figures 5-28, 5-29, 5-30, 5-56 to 5-75, 5-77 to 5-81, 5-103 to 5-110, 5-127 to 5-132, 5-154, 5-162, and 5-163). The most often proposed pathogenesis of ulcerative fungal keratitis in horses begins with slight to severe corneal trauma resulting in an epithelial defect, colonization of the defect by fungi normally present on the cornea, and subsequent stromal invasion. Seeding of fungi from a foreign body of plant origin is also possible. Some fungi may have the ability to invade the corneal epithelium following disruption of the tear film. A concurrent viral corneal infection may be present to weaken the corneal defense mechanisms.

✓ Stromal destruction results from the release of proteinases and other enzymes from the fungi, tear film leukocytes and keratocytes. Fungi may produce antiangiogenic compounds that inhibit vascularization.

✓ Fungi appear to have an affinity for Descemet's membrane with hyphae frequently found deep in the equine cornea. Deeper corneal invasion can lead to sterile or infectious endophthalmitis. Hyphae have been found in the posterior chamber three months following treatment for ulcerative keratomycosis.

✓ Saddlebreds appear to be prone to severe keratomycosis, while standardbreds are resistant.

☗ Diagnostic tests should include fluorescein and rose bengal staining, corneal cytology, corneal culture with attempted growth on both fungal and aerobic plates, and biopsy if surgery is performed.

✓ Prompt diagnosis and aggressive medical therapy with topically administered antifungals, antibiotics and atropine, and systemically administered NSAIDs will positively influence visual outcome, and may negate the need for surgical treatment.

☗ Treatment must be directed against the fungi as well as against the iridocyclitis that occurs following fungal replication and fungal death.

🗝 Therapy is quite prolonged and scarring of the cornea may be prominent.

🗝 The fungi are overall more susceptible to antifungal drugs in this order: natamycin = miconazole > itraconazole > ketoconazole > fluconazole.

✓ Natamycin, miconazole, itraconazole/DMSO, fluconazole, amphotericin B, povidone iodine solution, chlorhexidine gluconate, posaconazole, voriconazole, and silver sulfadiazine can be utilized topically singly or in combination.

🗝 **Uveitis may be worse the day following initiation of antifungal therapy due to fungal death.**

✓ Lufenuron is a chitin synthase inhibitor used orally to attack the fungal cell wall in horses with keratomycosis. Its efficacy needs to be determined.

✓ Systemically administered voriconazole, itraconazole or fluconazole may be useful in recalcitrant cases.

Iris Prolapse in the Horse

🗝 Iris prolapse (IP) in the horse most frequently follows acute sharp perforating corneal injuries (see Figure 5-11, 5-13, 5-14, 5-15, 5-17, 5-87, 5-121 and 5-135).

🗝 Corneal perforation can also occur secondary to rapid enzymatic degradation of stromal collagen and ground substance due to infectious and noninfectious ulcerative keratitis (see Figures 5-11, 5-14, 5-17 and 5-133 to 5-144).

✓ The eye may be cloudy, red, and painful. Blepharospasm and tearing are present.

✓ A brown to red colored structure protruding through a corneal or scleral laceration is diagnostic.

🗝 The anterior chamber will be shallow or collapsed due to loss of aqueous humor.

🗝 ◉ Fluorescein dye will indicate the site of a corneal perforation with a positive Seidel's test. The dye may also leak into the anterior chamber (Video 22).

✋ ◉ The indirect pupillary light reflex (PLR from the injured eye to the normal eye) should be utilized to determine if the damaged eye has the capability of vision (Video 9).

🗝 Horses presented with IP of fewer than 15 days duration, or horses with corneal lacerations and IP less than 15 mm in length, tend to have a favorable visual outcome.

☞ Keratomalacia, hyphema, corneal lacerations longer than 15 mm, and lacerations extending beyond the limbus adversely influence visual outcome.

✓ ⊙ Surgical repair should be attempted in all cases of IP. Topically applied antibiotics, atropine, and serum are recommended. Systemic NSAIDs and broad-spectrum parenteral antibiotics are also indicated (Video 20).

✓ Iridectomy does not appear to exacerbate anterior uveitis or adversely affect visual outcome.

✓ Ocular survival was 80% and 67% in horses with iris prolapse caused by corneal lacerations and melting ulcers, respectively. Vision may be retained in 40% of IP eyes.

Corneal Stromal Abscesses

✓ Corneal stromal abscesses can be a vision threatening sequelae to apparently minor corneal ulceration in the horse. A painful, blinding chronic iridocyclitis can result (Figures 5-168 to 5-243).

☞ Focal trauma to the cornea can inject microbes and debris into the corneal stroma through small epithelial ulcerative micropunctures (see Figures 5-168 to 5-171) and (Figure 5-244).

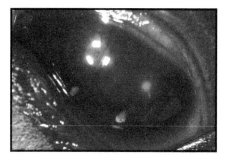 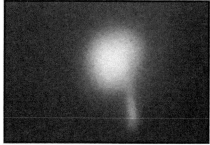

Figure 5-168 (left) A deep stromal abscess with a linear track to the corneal surface is found in a foal.

Figure 5-169 (right) Highly magnified image of the abscess and track in Figure 5-168. The track is <1mm long. The linear track was gone the next day.

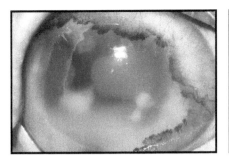
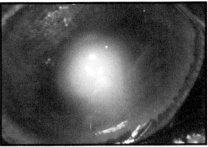

Figure 5-170 (left) Two deep stromal abscesses on the right are found with an iris abscess involving the corpora nigra on the left. The tips of the superficial corneal vessels are hemorrhaging into the stroma.

Figure 5-171 (right) A linear micropuncture track to the surface is present in this foal with a deep stromal abscess.

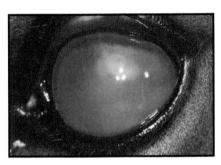
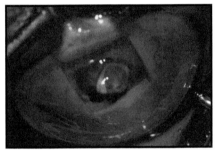

Figure 5-172 (left) Deep stromal abscess at the limbus has blood vessels moving towards it.

Figure 5-173 (right) Surgical removal of the abscess and corneal transplantation were used for therapy. This intraoperative photograph of Figure 5-172 reveals part of the abscess adhered to the iris.

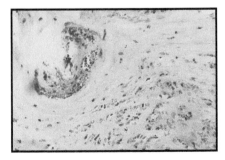
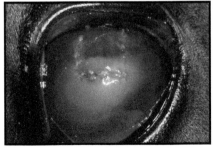

Figure 5-174 (left) Leukocytes and monocytes are present in the biopsy of the eye in Figure 5-172. H and E.

Figure 5-175 (right) The flap of cornea above the abscess in the eye in Figure 5-172 and corneal graft are healing.

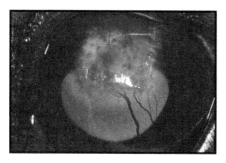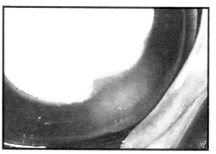

Figure 5-176 (left) The cornea has cleared and the graft healed one month after surgery in the eye in Figure 5-172.

Figure 5-177 (right) Deep stromal abscess near the limbus beneath superficial blood vessels.

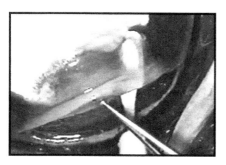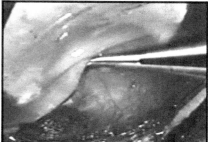

Figure 5-178 (left) A deep lamellar endothelial keratoplasty is used for therapy of the eye in Figure 5-177. The superficial cornea is incised to expose the abscess.

Figure 5-179 (right) The abscess is exposed and partially vascularized in the eye in Figure 5-177.

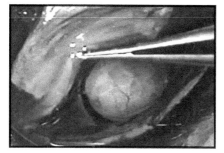

Figure 5-180 The stroma around the abscess has been incised in the eye in Figure 5-179.

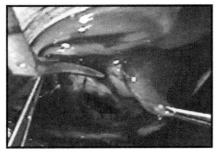
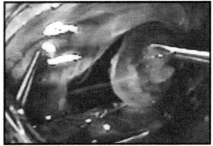

Figure 5-181 (left) Corneal scissors are used to remove the abscess in the eye in Figure 5-177. The white area beneath the abscess is fungus projecting into the anterior chamber.

Figure 5-182 (right) The abscess is removed in the eye in Figure 5-177. Brown iris is exposed.

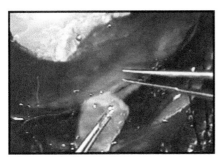
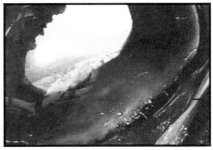

Figure 5-183 (left) A corneal graft is inserted in the defect and sutured in the abscess in the eye in Figure 5-177.

Figure 5-184 (right) The limbal incision is sutured in the eye in Figure 5-177. Some fibrin is near the pupil in the anterior chamber.

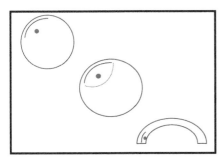
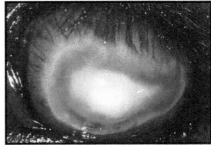

Figure 5-185 (left) This figure illustrates the surgery performed in Figure 5-177. The abscess is red. A limbal incision is made (upper left), the stroma is dissected to expose the abscess (middle), and the abscess exposed for removal (lower right).

Figure 5-186 (right) Large full thickness central stromal abscess with profound vascularization was treated medically.

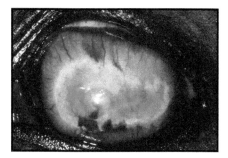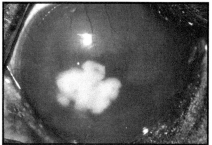

Figure 5-187 (left) Vascularization has healed the abscess in the eye in Figure 5-187 after two weeks with some limbal clearing of the cornea. The eye was comfortable but vision limited one month after.

Figure 5-188 (left) Large iris abscess due to fungus was associated mild uveitis.

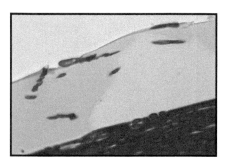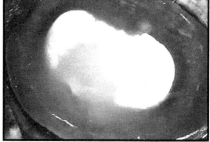

Figure 5-189 (right) Fungi invaded the lens capsule in the eye from Figure 5-188.

Figure 5-190 (right) Deep stromal abscess near the center of the cornea.

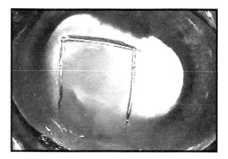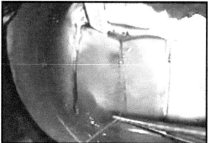

Figure 5-191 (left) A posterior lamellar keratoplasty and corneal transplant is utilized following medical therapy in the eye in Figure 5-190. A half thickness, three sided incision is made.

Figure 5-192 (right) Corneal dissectors are used to split the corneal thickness in the eye in Figure 5-190.

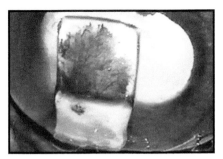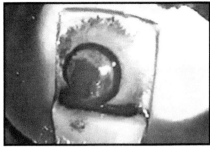

Figure 5-193 (left) The abscess in Figure 5-190 is exposed to reveal it is vascularized.

Figure 5-194 (right) A trephine outlines the abscess in Figure 5-190.

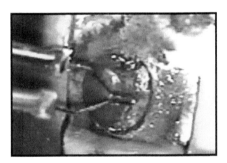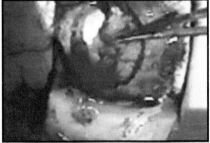

Figure 5-195 (left) Cautery is used to reduce hemorrhaging in the eye in Figure 5-190.

Figure 5-196 (right) The cornea is penetrated and the abscess removed in the eye in Figure 5-190.

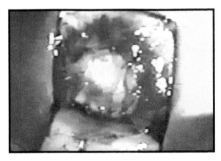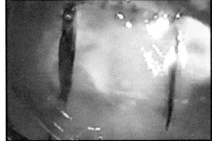

Figure 5-197 (left) A split thickness donor graft is placed and sutured in the eye in Figure 5-190.

Figure 5-198 (right) The superficial flap is sutured in the eye in Figure 5-190.

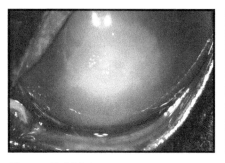 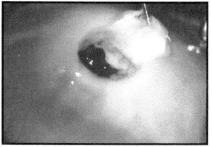

Figure 5-199 (left) Stromal abscess is near full thickness and associated with severe uveitis.

Figure 5-200 (right) Intraoperative photograph of the eye in Figure 5-199 shows the necrotic abscess touching the dark iris.

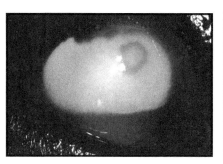 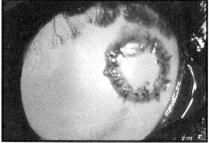

Figure 5-201 (left) Stromal abscess that had superficial and deep stromal involvement.

Figure 5-202 (right) Full thickness corneal transplant in the eye in Figure 5-201.

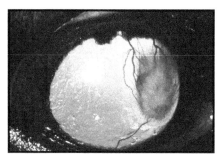 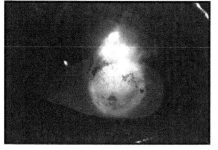

Figure 5-203 (left) Transplant is opaque 5.5 weeks after surgery in the eye in Figure 5-201.

Figure 5-204 (right) Transplant is slightly pigmented 1.2 years after surgery in the eye in Figure 5-201.

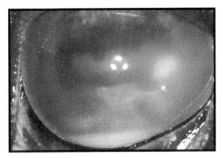 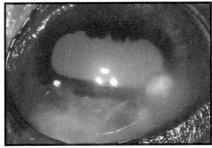

Figure 5-205 (left) Deep stromal abscess and hypopyon in a saddlebred gelding.

Figure 5-206 (right) Fibrin is organizing and the pupil slightly dilated after one day of medical therapy for the horse in Figure 5-205.

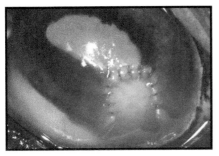 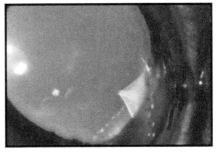

Figure 5-207 (left) PLK was performed for the abscess in Figure 5-205.

Figure 5-208 (right) The endothelium is coming off the donor graft and extending into the anterior chamber three days after PLK in the eye in Figure 5-205.

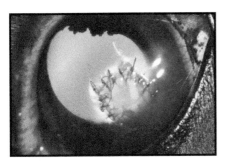 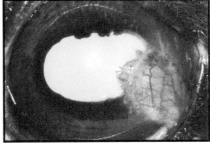

Figure 5-209 (left) Eight days post-PLK has some graft edema in the eye in Figure 5-205.

Figure 5-210 (right) A leak around the incision necessitated placement of a conjunctival flap which is adhered one month post PLK in the eye in Figure 5-205.

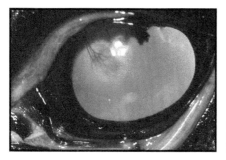
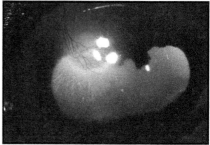

Figure 5-211 (left) Diffuse and deep stromal abscess is partially vascularized.

Figure 5-212 (right) The abscess is more white and healed after two weeks of medical therapy.

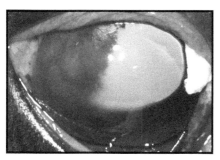
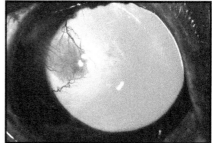

Figure 5-213 (left) Large stromal abscess is partially obscured by superficial vascularization.

Figure 5-214 (right) The abscess in Figure 5-213 has responded to medical therapy after two weeks of therapy.

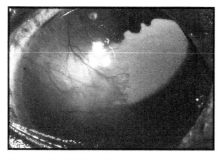
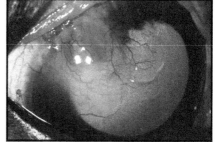

Figure 5-215 (left) Two deep stromal abscesses appear in the horse of Figure 5-213 two weeks after the eye in Figure 5-214.

Figure 5-216 (right) A DLEK procedure resolved the condition. Photograph was taken two months after the eye in Figure 5-215.

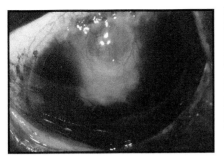 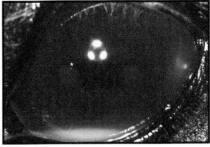

Figure 5-217 (left) The eye in Figure 5-215 2.5 months post-PLK.

Figure 5-218 (right) Deep stromal abscess obscured by blood vessels has a fluorescein positive track to the corneal surface. Hypopyon and miosis indicate uveitis.

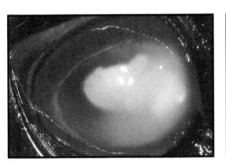 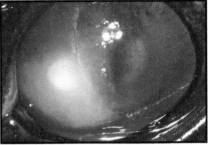

Figure 5-219 (left) Large stromal abscess has a track to the surface. Corneal edema and limbal vascularization are quite pronounced.

Figure 5-220 (right) Deep stromal abscess is nearly surrounded by blood vessels.

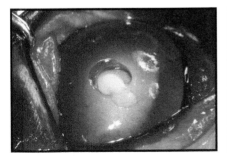 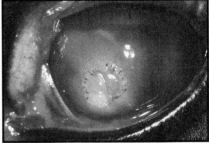

Figure 5-221 (left) A full thickness corneal transplant was performed. The white abscess protrudes into the anterior chamber in this intraoperative photo of the eye in Figure 5-220.

Figure 5-222 (right) A superficial ulcer is present three days after corneal transplantation in the eye in Figure 5-220.

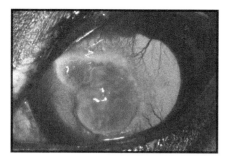 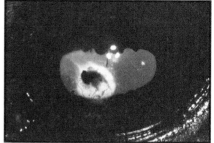

Figure 5-223 (left) Exuberant granulation tissue formed at the transplant site 6 weeks after surgery in the eye in Figure 5-220.

Figure 5-224 (right) A small opacity in the eye in Figure 5-223 is present two years post-transplantation in the eye in Figure 5-223.

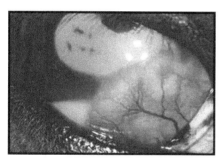 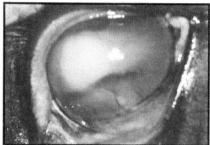

Figure 5-225 (left) Multiple stromal abscesses and severe uveitis are found in this eye. (From Adolfo Garcia).

Figure 5-226 (right) Extremely large deep stromal abscess is attracting superficial blood vessels.

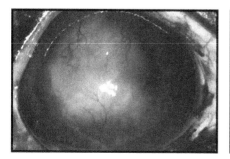 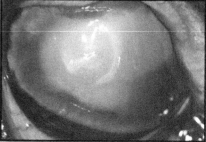

Figure 5-227 (left) The abscess is resolving after three weeks of medical therapy in the eye in Figure 5-226.

Figure 5-228 (right) Fusarium melting ulcer in a Hanoverian gelding.

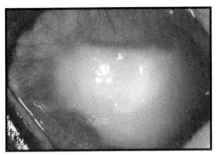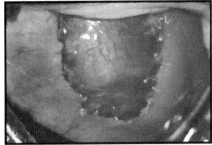

Figure 5-229 (left) The ulcerated area is more necrotic and forming an abscess after 13 days of medical therapy in the eye in Figure 5-228.

Figure 5-230 (right) A corneal transplant and conjunctival flap were used for therapy in the eye in Figure 5-229.

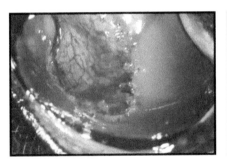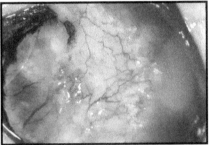

Figure 5-231 (left) The cornea is clearing four days after surgery in the eye in Figure 5-230.

Figure 5-232 (right) The conjunctival flap is pale and uveitis better nine days after the image in Figure 5-230.

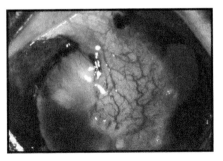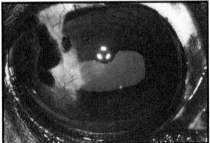

Figure 5-233 (left) The eye is much healthier and the eye visual 23 days after surgery in the eye in Figure 5-230.

Figure 5-234 (right) The eye in Figure 5-230 is in very good health 2 years later.

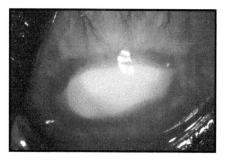 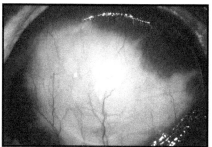

Figure 5-235 (left) Large stromal abscess obscured by superficial vessels in an Arabian filly.

Figure 5-236 (right) A generalized corneal scar is present after 41 days of medical therapy in the eye in Figure 5-235.

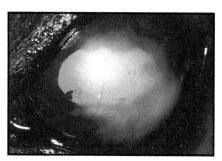 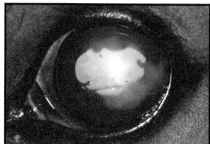

Figure 5-237 (left) The scarring resembles edema at 8 months after Figure 5-235. Some synechia are present.

Figure 5-238 (right) The eye in Figure 5-235 has some corneal opacity 3 years after the initial abscess.

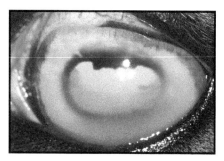 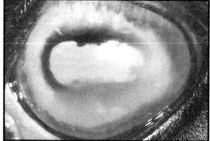

Figure 5-239 (left) Small white deep stromal abscess at the lateral limbus. Uveitis is causing corneal cloudiness.

Figure 5-240 (right) Seven days of medical therapy in the eye in Figure 5-239 have improved the uveitis slightly.

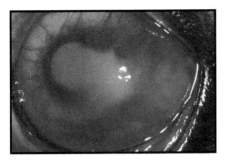 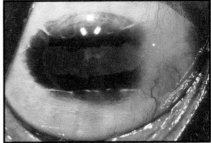

Figure 5-241 (left) Three weeks of medical therapy in the eye in Figure 5-239 demonstrate vascularization near the abscess.

Figure 5-242 (right) The abscess in Figure 5-239 is healed after two months of medical therapy. The iris color has returned to blue.

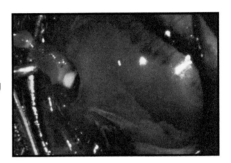

Figure 5-243 Deep stromal abscess has a white avascular portion projecting into the anterior chamber.

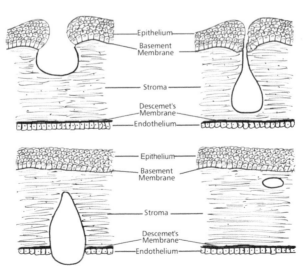

Figure 5-244 Stromal abscess therapy and prognosis depends on the type of abscess being treated. Most abscesses begin with as a micropuncture or a small corneal ulcer (upper left) that rapidly epithelializes (upper right) to cover a superficial or midstromal abscess (lower right), or a deep abscess (lower left).

🔑 A corneal abscess may develop after epithelial cells adjacent to the epithelial micropuncture divide and migrate over the small traumatic ulcer to encapsulate infectious agents or foreign bodies in the stroma. Epithelial cells are more likely to cover a fungal than a bacterial infection.

🔑 Reepithelialization forms a barrier that protects the bacteria or fungi from topically administered antimicrobial medications. Reepithelialization of stromal abscesses interferes with both routine diagnostics and treatment.

♥ Some stromal abscesses are definitely not related to superficial corneal trauma but appear to be associated with endothelial cell invasion by fungi or mycobaterial species. The mechanism for this is not understood, but clusters of cases suggest that more than traumatic etiologies are involved!! Recurrence of abscesses in the same eye also suggest a nontraumatic etiology. Some stromal abscesses may be ocular manifestations of a nondiagnosed systemic disease. Free floating "abscesses" have been noted with later stromal and iris attachment.

✓ Most stromal abscesses involving Descemet's membrane are fungal infections. The fungi seem "attracted" to the type IV collagen of Descemet's membrane, and may form "tunnels" using proteinases to the deeper stroma. Avascular tissue may be present in the anterior chamber.

🔑 Both superficial and deep stromal abscesses do not heal until they become vascularized. The patterns of corneal vascularization are often unique suggesting that vasoactive inhibitory factors released from the abscess influence the vascular response (see Figures 5-175, 5-187, 5-227, 5-236, 5-242) and (Figures 5-245 to 5-253).

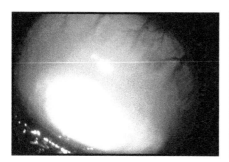 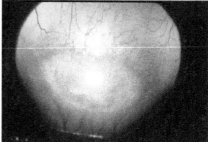

Figure 5-245 (left) Vascularization aids healing of a large superficial stromal abscess.

Figure 5-246 (right) An axial fibrovascular corneal scar is present in the horse in Figure 5-50 after 6 weeks of medical therapy.

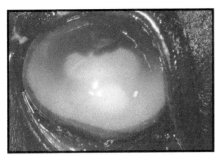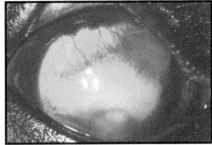

Figure 5-247 (left) An oval deep stromal abscess is found in the ventral cornea associated with hypopyon and anterior chamber fibrin.

Figure 5-248 (right) Corneal blood vessels remain superficial to the abscess after 11 days of medical therapy in the eye in Figure 5-247. Signs of uveitis are diminished.

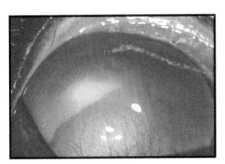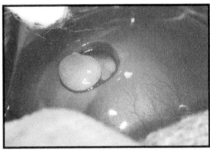

Figure 5-249 (left) A large diameter yellow stromal abscess is being covered by superficial vessels. Signs of uveitis are pronounced.

Figure 5-250 (right) Intraoperative photograph of a penetrating keratoplasty in the horse in Figure 5-249 demonstrates the deep nature of the abscess.

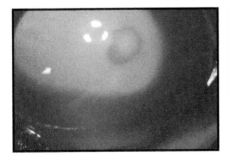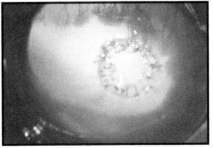

Figure 5-251 (left) Stromal abscess located deep in the cornea is caused by a fungus. Note the near absence of corneal vascularization in this case.

Figure 5-252 (right) One week following a penetrating keratoplasty for the stromal abscess in the eye in Figure 5-251. The eye is less inflamed, and the graft site displays corneal edema.

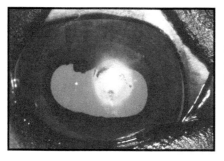

Figure 5-253 Fifteen months following the penetrating keratoplasty in the eye in Figure 5-251 a central scar is present. Vision is functionally normal and the eye is pain free.

✓ Medical therapy consists of aggressive use of topical and systemic antibiotics, topical atropine, and topical and systemic NSAIDs.

✓ Superficial stromal abscesses may initially respond positively to medical therapy. If reduced inflammation of the cornea and uvea are not found after two to three days of medical treatment, surgical removal of the abscess should be considered.

♥ Daily removal of superficial epithelium may speed drug penetration to a superficial abscess but probably does little for deeper abscesses. Aspiration of stromal abscesses is not recommended as the "abscess" material is rarely liquefied.

🔑 Deep posterior lamellar (PLK), deep endothelial lamellar (DLEK), and penetrating keratoplasties (PK) are three techniques of corneal transplantation used in the horse. PLK and DLEK are utilized in abscesses localized near Descemet's membrane with intrusion of the necrotic abscess into the anterior chamber. The superficial stroma is preserved in PLK and DLEK. PK is utilized for abscesses involving the entire corneal thickness. These techniques eliminate sequestered microbial antigens, and remove necrotic debris, cyotokines and toxins from degenerating leukocytes in the abscess.

✓ ⊙ **Posterior lamellar keratoplasty (PLK), Deep lamellar endothelial keratoplasty (DLEK), and Penetrating Keratoplasty for Deep Corneal Stromal Abscesses** (Videos 17-19 and 29).

✓ Corneal transplantation is performed to restore vision, to treat medically refractory corneal disease, and to replace damaged or missing corneal tissue.

🔑 Penetrating keratoplasty (PK),(see Figures 5-199, 5-229) posterior lamellar keratoplasty (PLK) (see Figures 5-190, 5-207) and (Figures 5-254 and 5-255), and deep lamellar endothelial keratoplasty (DLEK) (see Figures 5-178, 5-185, 5-216) are the types of corneal transplant procedures used in horses. All of these procedures have a high-risk for donor tissue rejection due to the fact that they are generally performed when corneal tissue is missing, or in infected or vascularized corneal tissue.

Penetrating keratoplasty is full thickness replacement of cornea in severe lacerations with iris prolapse, melting ulcers with impending iris prolapse, and full thickness stromal abscesses. Posterior lamellar keratoplasty and DLEK preserve the healthy anterior stroma when stromal abscesses with involvement of Descemet's membrane are excised and the tissue replaced with a partial thickness stroma/endothelial graft. PLK is used in central stromal abscesses and DLEK for stromal abscesses near the limbus.

✓ Fresh corneal grafts are preferred in horses, but frozen tissue can be utilized.

✓ Vascularization and edematous swelling of the donor grafts, indicating rejection, can be severe and begins at 5-10 days postoperatively.

⊶ Few equine PLK, DLEK, or PK grafts remain clear following their vascularization. They do perform very effective therapeutic and tectonic functions. Infectious endophthalmitis is a potential postoperative risk factor in a minority of cases.

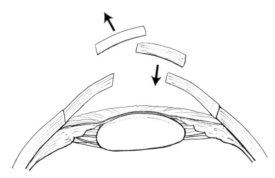

Figure 5-254 Penetrating keratoplasty (PK) involves the removal of a full thickness section of abnormal cornea and its replacement with a full thickness piece of normal donor cornea.

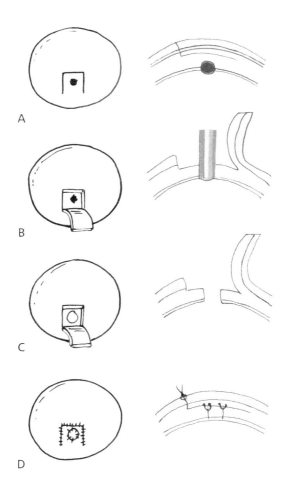

Figure 5-255 Posterior lamellar keratoplasty (PLK) is used for deep stromal abscesses where the cornea superficial to the abscess is not affected (A). The cornea superficial to the abscess is lifted to expose the abscess (B), the abscess is removed with a trephine (C), and the donor graft and superficial flap of cornea sutured in place (D).

Section 6

Other Corneal Problems

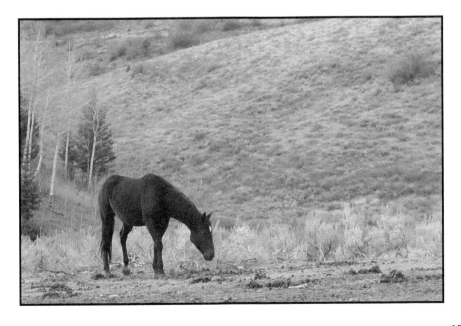

Corneal Edema

♥ The anterior half of the equine cornea is more hydrophilic than the posterior stroma such that edema is more prominent anteriorly. The epithelium of the horse cornea traps water to result in epithelial edema with bullae formation. Epithelial edema can double the thickness of the horse cornea.

♥ Corneal edema can be caused by ulcers or endothelial disease. The equine corneal endothelium does not appear to undergo mitosis.

♥ Vertical corneal edema can be an early sign of glaucoma in the horse (see Figure 7-62).

✓ Hypertonic solutions (5% sodium chloride) may be beneficial to remove edema. Thermatokeratoplasty may be necessary to reduce the edema in severe cases.

Squamous Cell Carcinoma and other Corneal Tumors

⛓ ⊙ Preneoplastic epithelial dysplasia, intraepithelial carcinoma in situ, and the invasive squamous cell carcinoma (SCC) are common to the limbus and cornea of horses (Figures 6-1 to 6-5). Epithelial dysplasia can be treated with topical 5-fluorouracil. Keratectomy and adjunctive therapies are needed for carcinoma in situ and SCC. Rapidly progressive and invasive SCC may necessitate enucleation (Figures 6-6 to 6-9) (Video 27).

✓ Limbal melanomas and hemangiosarcomas have also been reported (Figure 6-11).

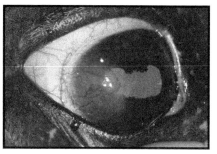 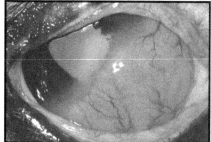

Figure 6-1 (left) Superficial nonulcerative keratitis with vascularization in an Arabian horse is epithelial dysplasia, a possible precursor to SCC. It was successfully treated with topical 5-FU.

Figure 6-2 (right) Limbal squamous cell carcinoma has extensively invaded the corneal stroma. The eye was enucleated.

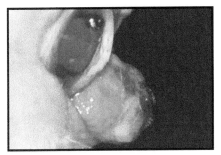 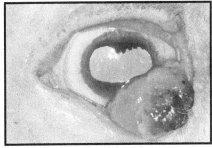

Figure 6-3 (left) Squamous cell carcinoma protrudes from the limbus.
Figure 6-4 (right) The tumor in Figure 6-3 has an ulcerated surface.

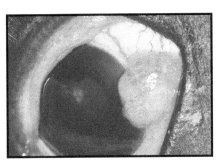 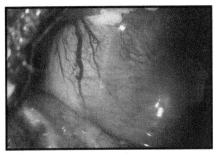

Figure 6-5 (left) Vascular squamous cell carcinoma of the limbus is present.
Figure 6-6 (right) Stromal Squamous cell carcinoma in a Belgian horse.

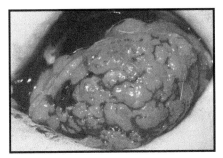 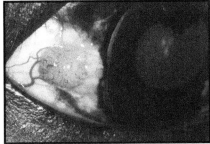

Figure 6-7 (left) Proliferative Squamous cell carcinoma of the cornea in a white horse.
Figure 6-8 (right) Limbal and conjunctival SCC in a horse.

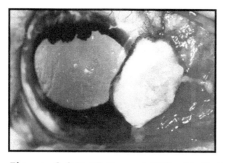 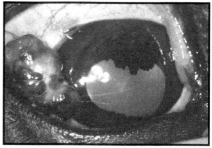

Figure 6-9 (left) Corneal SCC with limbal and conjunctival involvement in a horse.

Figure 6-10 (right) Limbal melanoma protrudes from the corneal surface.

Corneal Foreign Bodies

✓ ⊙ Penetrating and perforating corneal foreign bodies cause varying degrees of keratitis and uveitis and are common in horses. Superficial foreign bodies can be removed under topical anesthesia and the subsequent ulcer treated medically (Figures 6-11 to 6-20). Deep corneal and penetrating foreign bodies may cause severe uveitis/endophthalmitis and require more aggressive care (Video 21).

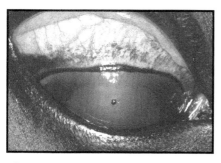 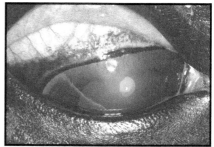

Figure 6-11 (left) A small corneal foreign body is adhered to the cornea.

Figure 6-12 (right) Removal of the foreign body in Figure 6-12 leaves a superficial corneal ulcer.

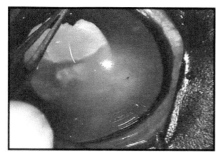

Figure 6-13 Small area of edema and large amount of fibrin in the anterior chamber of a horse with a "small" corneal foreign body.

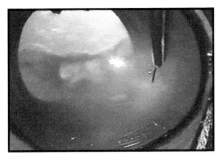
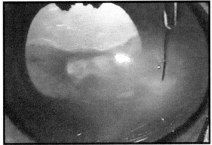

Figure 6-14 (left) Foreign body being removed with forceps in the eye in Figure 6-13.

Figure 6-15 (right) Foreign body in Figure 6-14 is quite large and removed. The corneal fistula was then sutured.

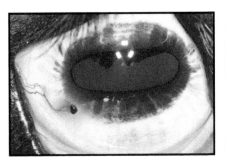
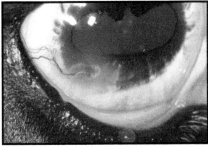

Figure 6-16 (left) This small brown foreign body is causing slight pain and induced vascularization.

Figure 6-17 (right) Gentle foreign body removal reveals a small corneal ulcer which healed rapidly in the eye in Figure 6-16.

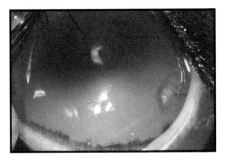
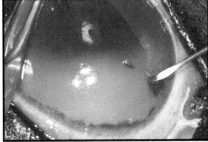

Figure 6-18 (left) An epithelial inclusion cyst and corneal edema in this horse.

Figure 6-19 (right) The cyst was formed by a grass foreign body in the eye in Figure 6-18.

Endothelial Detachment following Blunt Trauma

✓ Profound and persistent corneal edema may be present following blunt trauma to the globe of the horse (Figure 6-20). Detachment of the endothelium is a proposed mechanism of this syndrome. The prognosis for a return to normal is poor. Hypertonic solutions (5% sodium chloride) may be beneficial in the early stages. Thermatokeratoplasty may be necessary to reduce the edema in severe cases. Endothelial cell reattachment and cellular hypertrophy can occur to resolve the condition in some horses.

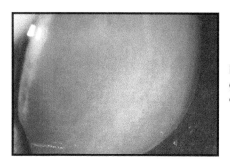

Figure 6-20 Blunt trauma to the globe resulted in acute generalized corneal edema.

Nonulcerative Keratouveitis (NKU)

✓ Nonulcerative keratouveitis (NKU) is characterized by a nonulcerated, fleshy, paralimbal corneal stromal infiltrate combined with a pronounced anterior uveitis. It is probably immune-mediated (sse Figure 6-23).

✓ Topical corticosteroids (1% prednisolone acetate or 0.1% dexamethasone 4 to 6 times daily), cyclosporine A (BID to TID), and mydriatics/cycloplegics (1% atropine SID to QID), with systemic nonsteroidal antiinflammatory drugs are indicated.

☞ Persistent, painful uveitis is severe with NKU and often results in enucleation due to intractable pain.

Nonulcerative Interstitial Keratitis (NIK)

♥ Several forms of NIK are found in Europe (Figures 6-21 to 6-26). Some are associated with a "history of ocular trauma". The etiology is presumed to be altered corneal immune privilege from abnormal exposure or expression of corneal antigens inducing autoimmune dysregulation. Nonulcerative superficial and nonulcerative recurrent forms of stromal keratitis are two types of NIK noted in European warmbloods. Stromal pigmentation and/or a greenish yellow stromal discoloration may occur in some eyes. An endotheliitis with slight to severe corneal edema is another form of NIK. These eyes may partially respond to topically administered corticosteroids, NSAIDs, tacrolimus or cyclosporine A, and may require parenteral antibiotics, corticosteroids, or NSAIDs. Endotheliitis may be found with lens subluxations.

♥ Limbal keratitis may occur in foals with placentitis.

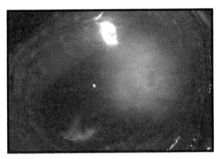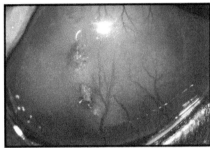

Figure 6-21 (left) Nonulcerative stromal keratitis in a horse from Florida.
Figure 6-22 (right) Nonulcerative stromal keratitis in a horse from Florida. The stroma was yellow green. The sutures are from corneal biopsies.

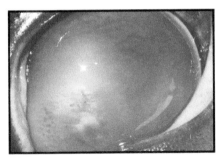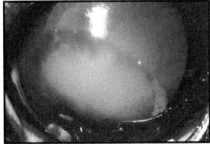

Figure 6-23 (left) Nonulcerative stromal keratopathy in a Quaterhorse resolved with topical erthromycin.
Figure 6-24 (right) Nonulcerative stromal keratopathy has stromal hemorrhage.

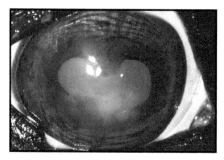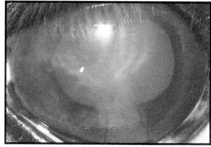

Figure 6-25 (left) Nonulcerative stromal keratopathy appears as multiple discrete foci.

Figure 6-26 (right) Nonulcerative stromal keratopathy is diffuse with superficial vessels in this eye.

Eosinophilic Keratoconjunctivitis

✓ Eosinophilic keratoconjunctivitis resembles a corneal tumor in appearance. Eosinophilic keratoconjunctivitis has an unknown etiology, but may be an immune-mediated disease. Horses living in the Ohio River Valley region are at risk. Horses with lengthy turnout times are most commonly affected.

✓ All ages and breeds of horses can be affected with many cases reported in the spring.

✓ Clinical signs include corneal granulation tissue, blepharospasm, chemosis, conjunctival hyperemia, mucoid discharge, and corneal ulcers covered by raised, white, necrotic plaques (Figures 6-28 to 6-33).

✓ KCS may develop in affected horses due to lacrimal gland inflammation. The lacrimal gland should be palpated to detect swelling.

✓ Corneal cytology typically contains numerous eosinophils and a few mast cells to rule out similar appearing infectious and neoplastic causes.

✓ Superficial lamellar keratectomy to remove large plaques speeds corneal healing.

℞ Topical corticosteroids (1% prednisolone acetate or 0.1% dexamethasone) 4 to 6 times a day in early stages (in spite corneal ulcerations), antibiotics (e.g., bacitracin-neomycin-polymyxin or tobramycin), 1% atropine, and 0.03% phospholine iodide (BID) in combination with systemic nonsteroidal antiinflammatory drugs are indicated. Topical cromolyn sodium (4.0% TID) or lodoxamide (0.1% TID), mast cell stabilizers, can also aid healing. Systemic corticosteroids may be necessary.

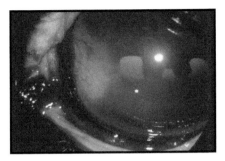
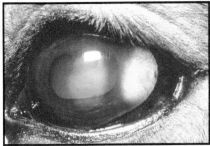

Figure 6-27 (left) The pink, fleshy, limbal lesion with miosis in this eye is characteristic of an immune-mediated condition called nonulcerative keratopathy.

Figure 6-28 (right) Lesions characteristic of eosinophilic keratitis are near the limbus.

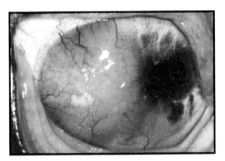
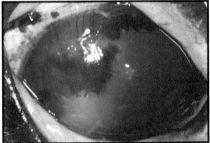

Figure 6-29 (left) Proliferative eosinophilic keratitis in a horse.

Figure 6-30 (right) Stromal hemorrhage and eosinophilic keratitis in a horse.

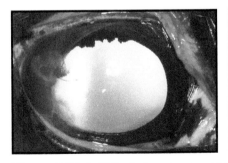
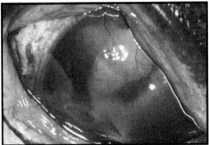

Figure 6-31 (left) Topical corticosteroid therapy has reduced the lesion size ten days later in the horse in Figure 6-30.

Figure 6-32 (right) The lesion is more opaque after 17 days of topical corticosteroid therapy in the horse in Figure 6-30.

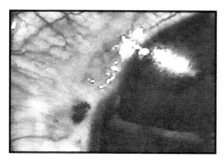

Figure 6-33 Intraoperative photograph of limbal and conjunctival eosinophilic keratitis in a horse. The lesions were considered more likely to be SCC prior to surgery.

✔ Horses should be dewormed twice with ivermectin 10 days apart. Switching to moxidectin may also be beneficial.

✔ These lesions are typically slow to heal. Scarring of the cornea occurs.

♥ Recurrence is possible, but reduced by limiting turnout times, and wearing a soft fly mask when turned out.

Herpes and Viral Keratitis

✔ Multiple, superficial, white, punctate or linear opacities of the cornea, with or without fluorescein dye retention, are found associated with equine herpes virus 2 and other viruses.

✔ The focal punctate corneal opacities may be found at the end of superficial corneal vessels, and may retain rose bengal stain. (figures 6-34 to 6-42)

✔ Varying amounts of ocular pain, conjunctivitis, and iridocyclitis are present.

✔ Multiple foals in a herd may be affected.

✔ Topically administered idoxuridine and trifluorothymidine (TID) have been used with topical NSAIDs for treatment of equine herpes ulcers, but recurrence is common.

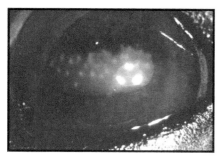

Figure 6-34 Multifocal white lesions are typical of herpes keratitis. They can stain intermittently with fluorescein and rose bengal.

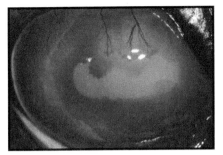 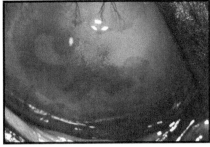

Figure 6-35 (left) Suspected viral keratitis with mild pain, generalized slight corneal edema and sparse superficial vascularization in German Warmblood stallion.

Figure 6-36 (right) Rose bengal retention in the eye in Figure 6-35.

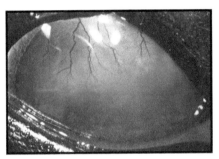 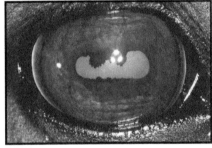

Figure 6-37 (left) The eye in Figure 6-35 1.5 years later. Various antiviral medications had been used unsuccessfully.

Figure 6-38 (right) The eye in Figure 6-37 14 months later. Intermittent topical NSAID use resolved the condition.

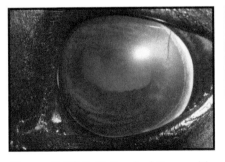 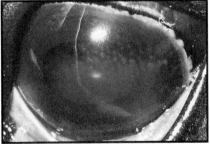

Figure 6-39 (left) Focal white opacities and sparse superficial vascularization suggest a viral keratitis in a horse from the UK. (From Andy Matthews).

Figure 6-40 (right) Multiple white opacities suggest a viral keratitis in this horse from Canada.

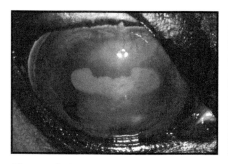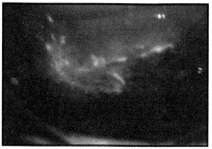

Figure 6-41 (left) Generalized corneal opacity and sparse superficial vascularization suggest a viral or immune mediated etiology in this Arab stallion from the northern USA.

Figure 6-42 (right) Acyclovir responsive superficial keratitis in this horse from Italy. (From Adolfo Guandalini).

Burdock Pappus Bristle Keratopathy

✂ Burdock pappus (*Arctium* spp) bristles are common conjunctival foreign bodies in the northeastern United States that can lead to chronic nonhealing corneal ulcers.

✓ Unilateral ocular signs include blepharospasm, serous or mucopurulent ocular discharge, and a positive corneal fluorescein dye uptake. The nictitans is commonly involved.

✓ Chronic epithelial erosion or ulceration can develop.

♥ Differential diagnoses include lid abnormalities such as ectopic cilia, distichiasis, trichiasis, and entropion; neuroparalytic and neurotrophic keratitis; keratoconjunctivitis sicca; infection, and corneal foreign bodies.

✓ Conjunctivalectomy and/or conjunctival debridement of the bristle foreign body and surrounding conjunctival tissue is required under sedation and auriculopalpebral nerve block. After conjunctivalectomy, topical antibiotics and atropine, and systemic phenylbutazone are used.

✓ Healing of the corneal defect occurs within three to 14 days after removal of the bristle.

Calcific Band Keratopathy

✓ Calcific band keratopathy (CBK) is a complication of chronic uveitis and consists of deposition of dystrophic calcium in the superficial corneal epithelium and stroma.

✓ Dense, white bands of calcium are noted in the interpalpebral region of the central cornea. (Figures 6-43 to 6-47).

✓ Scattered areas of fluorescein retention are present as the calcium disrupts the epithelium to result in painful superficial ulcers. Deep ulcers can develop.

✓ A gritty sensation is found durinq scraping for corneal cytology.

☞ It appears to develop in the eyes of horses most aggressively treated with topical corticosteroids for ERU. CBK is rare in ERU horses that have not been treated medically!

✓ Treatment is topically administered calcium chelaters (dipotassium ethylene diamine tetraacetate 1%, Sequester-Sol®) to decrease tear calcium levels and aid healing.

✓ Topical antibiotics, atropine, and systemic non-steroidal anti-inflammatory drugs are also beneficial for the ulcers.

✓ Superficial keratectomy may be necessary to remove the painful calcium deposits.

♥ Healing of keratectomy sites can occur with severe scarring.

♥ Recurrence of calcium band keratopathy is possible with continued episodes of uveitis. The prognosis for vision is guarded because of subsequent corneal scarring and further uveitis episodes.

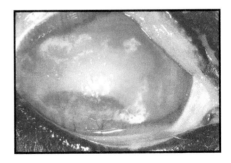

Figure 6-43 White calcium deposits causing ulceration and vascularization of the cornea in a horse with chronic uveitis induced band keratopathy.

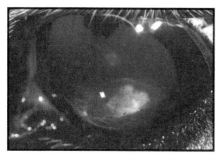
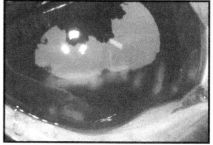

Figure 6-44 (left) White calcium deposits in an ERU eye.

Figure 6-45 (right) Calcium deposits associated with band keratopathy in an eye with chronic ERU have caused multiple ulcers.

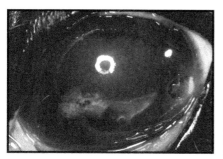
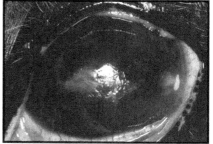

Figure 6-46 (left) Fluorescein positive areas of calcium deposition in an eye with ERU.

Figure 6-47 (right) The corneal surface appears dry in the eye in Figure 6-46.

Section 7

Cataracts, Glaucoma and Uveal Problems in the Horse

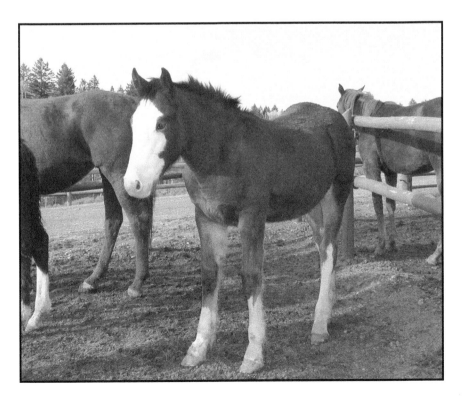

Cataracts

✓ Cataracts are opacities of the lens and are a frequent congenital ocular defect in foals (see Figure 2-54) and (Figures 7-1 to 7-16).

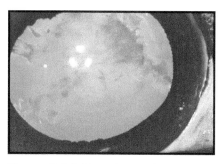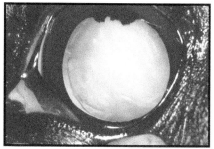

Figure 7-1 (left) Nuclear and some cortical cataractous changes in the lens of a foal.
Figure 7-2 (right) Immature cataract in a foal.

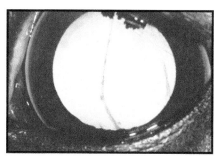

Figure 7-3 The eye in Figure 7-2 6 days after cataract surgery is clear with tears in the anterior and posterior capsules evident.

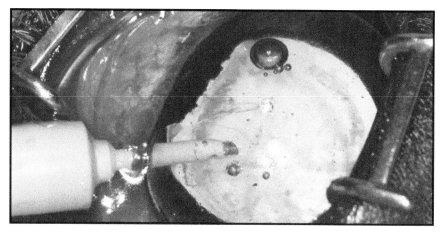

Figure 7-4 Intraoperative photograph of phacoemulsification cataract surgery in a foal.

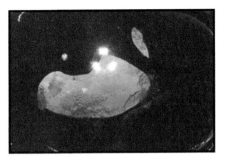 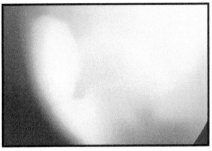

Figure 7-5 (left) Posterior and anterior capsular opacification have severely limited vision in the eye in Figure 7-4 although the surgery was technically successful.

Figure 7-6 (right) Large pieces of lens cortex are found sitting on the retina from a spontaneous lens capsule rupture prior to cataract surgery.

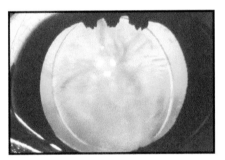 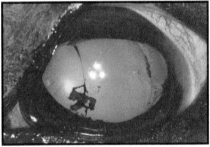

Figure 7-7 (left) An immature cataract in the adult horse in Figure 7-6.

Figure 7-8 (right) Traumatic lens luxation in a horse.

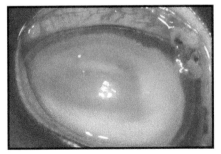 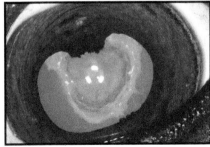

Figure 7-9 (left) Endophthalmitis 10 days following seemingly unremarkable cataract surgery was treated by enucleation.

Figure 7-10 (right) Nuclear cataract in an adult horse.

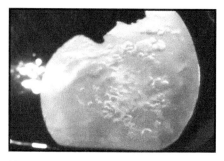 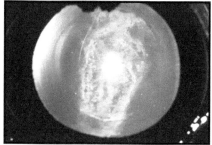

Figure 7-11 (left) Cortical and nuclear vacuoles are swollen lens fibers in a Thoroughbred stallion with uveitis.

Figure 7-12 (right) Nuclear and cortical cataract in an adult horse. A perinuclear halo is also present.

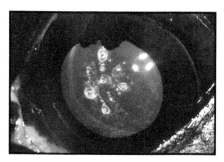 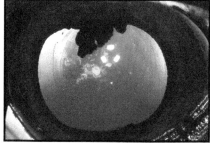

Figure 7-13 (left) Several focal nuclear cataracts in an adult horse.

Figure 7-14 (right) Focal nuclear opacities and a perinuclear halo in an adult horse.

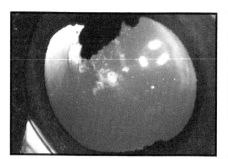 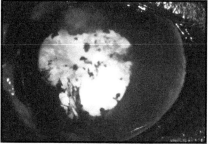

Figure 7-15 (left) Different angle of illuminating light illustrates focal cataracts in Figure 7-14.

Figure 7-16 (right) Extensive posterior synechiation and cataract formation in a horse with ERU.

♥ Horses manifest varying degrees of blindness as cataracts mature. Very small incipient lens opacities are common and not associated with blindness. Cataracts of the anterior lens can progress while cataracts of the posterior lens and nucleus do not.

⚲ As cataracts mature and become more opaque, the degree of blindness increases. The tapetal reflection is seen with incipient and immature cataracts, but is not seen in mature cataracts. Lens dislocation or luxation may also occur with cataracts in horses (Figures 7-17 to 7-19). Lens cysts may be noticed in a few cases (Figures 7-20 to 7-24).

✓ Examination of the fundus may be difficult due to the cataract. The rate of cataract progression and development of blindness cannot be predicted in most instances.

⚲ The basic mechanism of cataract formation is a decrease in soluble lens proteins, failure of the lens epithelial cell sodium pump, a decrease in lens glutathione, and lens fiber swelling and fiber membrane rupture.

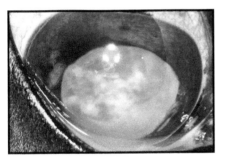 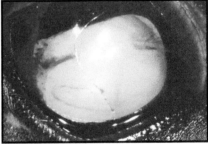

Figure 7-17 (left) Anteriorly luxated cataract in an old horse.

Figure 7-18 (right) Resolving hyphema from ocular trauma in a horse. An aphakic crescent is noted at the 1 to 3 o'clock position of the pupil.

Figure 7-19 The luxated lens is becoming cataractous four weeks later in the eye in Figure 7-18. Corneal opacity is related to tension caused by the resorbing blood clot.

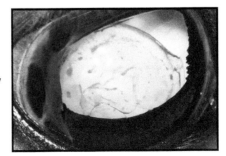

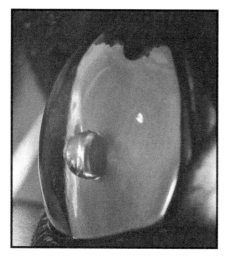

Figure 7-20 Lens cyst protrudes anteriorly from the lens capsule in an Arabian stallion.

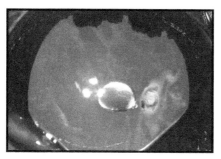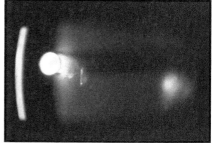

Figure 7-21 (left) A small cataract is to the right of the lens cyst in Figure 7-20. It was noted to progress in size over a two month period.

Figure 7-22 (right) Slitlamp view of shadow produced by the lens cyst. The horse overreacted to movements near this eye due to shadow movements on the retina. Removal of the lens corrected the behavioral problem.

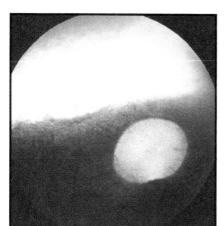

Figure 7-23 Focal tapetal retinal lesion in the horse in Figure 7-20 was not present preoperatively and may have been caused by phototoxicity from the operating microscope light.

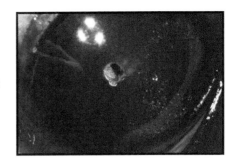

Figure 7-24 Focal lens cyst in an older Thoroughbred mare. There was no effect on vision.

🗝 Heritable, traumatic, nutritional, and postinflammatory etiologies have been proposed for equine cataracts. Cataracts secondary to equine recurrent uveitis (ERU) or trauma are frequently seen in adults. EPM is a reported cause of unilateral cataracts. True senile cataracts that interfere with vision are found in horses older than 20 years. Hypermature cataracts may become intumescent again in thoroughbreds.

✓ Increased cloudiness of the lens occurs with age and is called nuclear sclerosis.(Figure 7-25) It is common in older horses, but vision is clinically normal, as nuclear sclerosis does not cause vision loss.

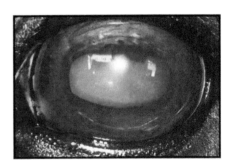

Figure 7-25 Nuclear sclerosis is an age related clouding of the lens. It may be mistaken for a cataract but is not associated with blindness as are cataracts.

Equine Cataract Surgery

🗝 ⊙ Most veterinary ophthalmologists recommend surgical removal of cataracts in foals less than 6 months of age if the foal is healthy, no uveitis or other ocular problems are present, and the foal's personality will tolerate aggressive topical medical therapy (Video 3). Opacification of the capsule occurs early in foals with cataracts.

✓ Horses considered for lens extraction should be in good physical condition. Complete ophthalmic and general physical examinations should be performed.

✓ Examine foals for subclinical Rhodococcus pneumonia and if present treat it prior to surgery.

✓ Adult horses with visual impairment due to cataracts are also candidates for cataract surgery. Posterior lens cataracts in immature stages of development appear to have the most effect on vision.

🖐 Slow or absent pupillary light reflexes (PLRs) may indicate active iridocyclitis with or without posterior synechiation, retinal disease, optic nerve disease, or iris sphincter muscle atrophy.

🔑 Afferent pupillary defects in a cataractous eye cannot be attributed to the cataract alone, as well as the fact that normal PLRs do not exclude some degree of retinal or optic nerve disease.

🔑 Any signs of inflammatory eyelid, conjunctival, or corneal disease, and anterior uveitis should delay cataract surgery until the inflammation has been successfully treated.

♥ ⊙ B-scan ultrasound and electroretinography are beneficial in assessing the anatomic and functional status of the retina if a cataract is present (Video 28).

🖐 General anesthesia with its attendant risks is required for cataract surgery.

Extracapsular Cataract Surgery

✓ A large clear corneal incision adjacent to the limbus is made for 180° around the circumference of the cornea. The anterior lens capsule is torn and removed with lens capsule forceps, and the lens nucleus and cortex gently expressed. The thin posterior lens capsule is left intact as a barrier to anterior vitreous movement and infection. Simple interrupted or simple continuous suture patterns of 7-0 absorbable suture are used to close the corneal wound. Irrigation/aspiration with lactated Ringer's solution containing heparin (2 IU/ml) is utilized to remove any remaining cortex.

Phacoemulsification Cataract Surgery

🔑 ⊙ This is the most useful technique for the horse (see Figures 2-54, 2-55) and (Figures 7-26 to 7-32) (Video 3). This extracapsular procedure through a 3.2mm corneal incision utilizes a piezoelectric handpiece with an ultrasonic titanium needle in a silicone sleeve to fragment and emulsify the lens nucleus and cortex following removal of the anterior capsule. The emulsified lens is then aspirated from the eye while intraocular pressure is maintained by infusion of lactated Ringer's solution containing epinephrine (1:10,000) and heparin (2 IU/ml) (see Figure 7-4) and (Video 3).

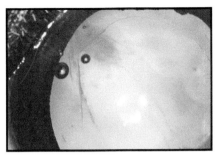
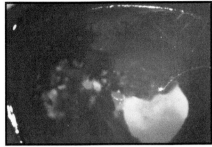

Figure 7-26 (left) Successful phacoemulsification cataract extraction in the horse in Figure 2-54.

Figure 7-27 (right) Persistent low level uveitis two years postoperatively in Figure 2-54 caused posterior synechiation and miotic pupil. Functional vision is present.

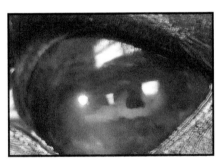
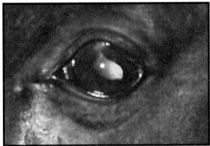

Figure 7-28 (left) Miosis, posterior synechiation and cataract formation in a 25 year old pony mare with ERU and cataract.

Figure 7-29 (right) Successful phacoemulsification cataract surgery in the eye in Figure 7-28 restored some vision. Note bright tapetal reflection.

Figure 7-30 Ultrasound of Figure 2-55 (cornea to the left) reveals a small cataract and normal retinal position (to the right).

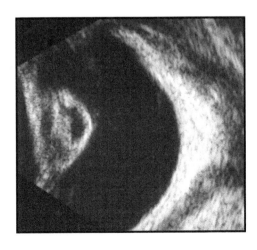

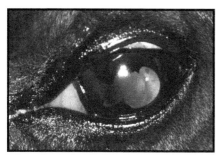 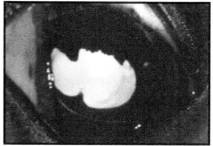

Figure 7-31 (left) Postoperative phacoemulsification photograph of the horse in Figure 2-55. Slight hyphema is present nasally.

Figure 7-32 (right) The cornea is clear and the foal in Figure 2-55 visual twenty six days postoperatively.

The globe is entered dorsally through a scleral tunnel under a limbal based conjunctival flap The keratome blade is entered to one side of the corpora nigra, as the corpora nigra can hemorrhage quite severely if touched, especially in adults. Trypan blue is injected to stain and visualize the anterior lens capsule. A 10 mm diameter piece of anterior capsule is removed. The anterior capsule may become opaque intraoperatively or days later in some foals.

The phaco tip is kept in the anterior chamber and the tip not angled posteriorly. The posterior capsule can rapidly move anteriorly and posteriorly when the eye is open in horses, although the vitreous is well formed and generally not liquefied. The equine posterior capsule tears quite easily. A 30 degree phaco needle can minimize tears in the posterior capsule. The viscous lens cortex of foals can often be aspirated through the 0.4 mm aspiration needle. Larger cataract pieces may only pass through the 0.9 mm diameter phaco needle. The elbows should be rested and the bursts of phaco power used to aspirate lens cortex to the phaco needle. Viscoelastic can be used to move large pieces of the lens to the phaco needle.

The surgeon may note retinal folds intraoperatively due to the low IOP that disappears later. The foal tapetum may appear "granular" intraoperatively and normal later.

Spontaneous rupture of the posterior capsule, posterior capsular cysts, and large anterior vitreal opacities are found in horses with cataracts (see Figures 7-20 to 7-24).

The cornea near the incision becomes cloudy for several days. There is little inflammation postoperatively in most horses. Flare, if present at all, clears in days. Hyphema can be a major problem if extensive. Foals regain sight quickly. Retinal detachment can occur in 48 hrs. The anterior chamber is shallow for 3-5 days postoperatively with the posterior capsule bulging forward.

✓ The thin posterior capsule is left intact. following phacoemulsification cataract surgery. There is a quicker return to normal activity with phacoemulsification than other surgical techniques.

Intracapsular Cataract Surgery

✓ In this technique, the lens is removed within the intact lens capsule. This technique is utilized for lens luxation with often poor results in the horse, and is thus not indicated for routine lens removal.

Postoperative Cataract Surgery Therapy and Results

✓ Topically applied antibiotics, such as chloramphenicol, gentamicin, ciprofloxacin, or tobramycin ophthalmic solutions may be utilized pre- and postoperatively. Frequency of medication varies from q2h to q8h.

✓ Topically applied 1 to 2 percent atropine is effective in stabilizing the blood-aqueous barrier, minimizing pain from ciliary muscle spasm, and causes pupillary dilatation. Atropine may be used as often as q4h, with the frequency of administration reduced as soon as the pupil dilates.

⚷ Topically applied corticosteroids, such as prednisolone acetate (1%), are essential to suppress pre- and postoperative inflammation.

✓ Systemically administered NSAIDs can be used orally or parenterally, and are effective in reducing anterior uveitis in horses with cataracts.

✓ Topically administered NSAIDs such as diclofenac, flurbiprofen and suprofen must also be used to suppress signs of anterior uveitis.

⚷ The results of cataract surgery in foals by experienced veterinary ophthalmologists are generally very good, but the cataract surgical results in adult horses with cataracts caused by ERU are often poor. The problem is that new blood vessels form on the iris and anterior lens capsule in the eyes with ERU and they can bleed during the surgeries. The surgeon often cannot stop the hemorrhage and severe hyphema results.

✓ Postoperative complications include persistent iridocyclitis and plasmoid aqueous, fibropupillary membranes, synechiae, corneal ulceration, corneal edema, posterior capsular opacification, retained lens cortex, wound leakage, vitreous presentation into anterior chamber, retinal detachment, and infectious endophthalmitis (see Figures 7-9, 7-27) and (Figures 7-33, 7-34).

🔑 Persistent corneal edema is the most common postoperative complication in adult horses with cataracts caused by uveitis. Posterior capsular opacification can be severe. Cataract surgery can be beneficial in the uveitic horse but does not cure the uveitis which will still be a problem.

🔑 Slight corneal edema is usually present from 24 to 72 hours postoperatively. One week following surgery the pupil should be functional, any fibrin in the anterior chamber resorbing, and the fundus visible. Three weeks following surgery the eye should be nonpainful, the patient visual, pupillary movement normal, and the ocular media clear.

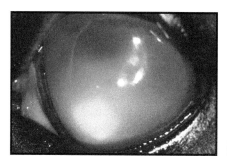 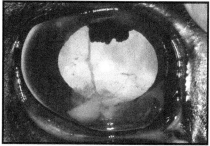

Figure 7-33 (left) A stromal abscess developed 33 days postoperatively in the eye in Figure 2-55. The abscess healed but vision was lost.

Figure 7-34 (right) Cataractous lens fragments remain in the anterior chamber after complicated phacoemulsification cataract surgery.

Aphakic Vision in Horses

🔑 Most reliable reports of vision in successful cataract surgery in horses indicate vision is functionally normal postoperatively. From an optical standpoint, the aphakic eye should be quite far-sighted or hyperopic postoperatively, and was +9.94D hyperopic in one study. Images close to the eye would be blurry and appear magnified.

🔑 The loss of accommodation could be severely debilitating to some horses. Theoretically, intraocular lenses (IOL) should improve post-operative visual outcome in horses. IOL refractive power of 25D resulted in +8D hyperopia by retinoscopy in one 1996 study of pseudophakic horses. A new foldable +14 D IOL resulted in +2.5 hyperopia in the pseudophakic eye in a 2007 study (Figure 7-35). A 30D IOL should allow emmetropica to be reached in the aphakic horse eye in a 2006 study.

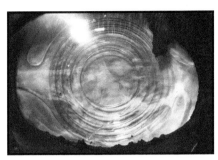

Figure 7-35 Intraocular lens placed after cataract removal in a horse.

Equine Glaucomas

✓ The glaucomas are a group of diseases resulting from alterations of aqueous humor dynamics that cause an intraocular pressure (IOP) increase above that which is compatible with normal function of the retinal ganglion cells and optic nerve.

☞ The **intraocular pressure (IOP)** of horses is 16-30 mm Hg with a Tonopen applanation tonometer (see Figure 2-17).

☞ Horses with previous or concurrent uveitis, aged horses, and Appaloosas are at increased risk for the development of glaucoma. Glaucoma has also been reported in the Quarter Horse, Tennessee Walking Horse, Thoroughbred, Arabian, Welsh pony, American Saddlebred, and warm bloods.

✓ The iridocorneal angle of horses should be monitored. It becomes more solid in horses with ERU. The angle may partially collapse but leave no other anterior segment changes in eyes that have had ocular trauma.

✓ Iris and ciliary body neoplasms can cause secondary glaucoma.

✓ Congenital glaucoma is reported in foals and associated with developmental anomalies of the iridocorneal angle.

✓ The infrequency of diagnosis in the horse may be due, in part, to the limited availability of tonometers in equine practice, but also to the fact that large fluctuations in intraocular pressure (IOP), even in chronic cases, may make documentation of elevated IOP difficult.

✓ Afferent pupillary light reflex deficits, corneal striae, corneal edema, decreased vision, lens luxations, mild iridocyclitis, and optic nerve atrophy/cupping may also be found in eyes of horses with glaucoma (Figures 7-36 to 7-66). Stria or band opacities are also found in normal horse eyes, but branch more in eyes with glaucoma.

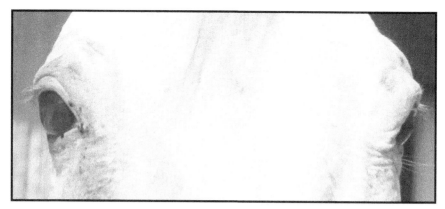

Figure 7-36 The right eye is buphthalmic and the cornea edematous in a horse with glaucoma.

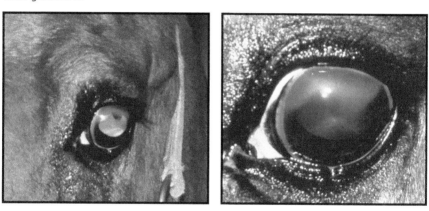

Figure 7-37 (left) Corneal edema in the dorsal region, mydriasis, and a linear opacity are present in the left eye of a horse with glaucoma.

Figure 7-38 (right) Close-up of the eye of the horse in Figure 7-37.

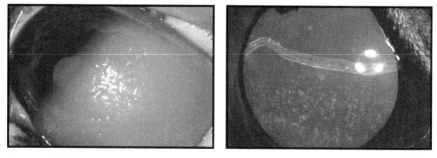

Figure 7-39 (left) Severe corneal edema with epithelial bullae formation in a horse with glaucoma.

Figure 7-40 (right) A thick corneal band opacity is found in some normal horses and in horses with glaucoma.

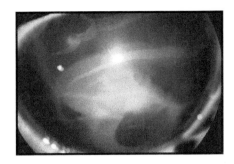

Figure 7-41 Branching stria and a luxated cataract in a horse with glaucoma.

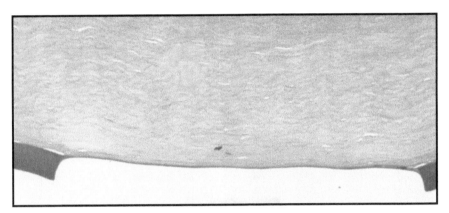

Figure 7-42 Histology of the stria from the horse in Figure 7-37 demonstrates a severe thinning, rather than rupture, of Descemet's membrane.

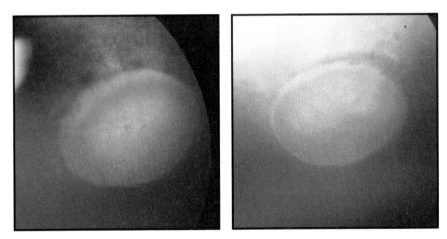

Figure 7-43 (left) Normal optic nerve of the right eye of the horse in Figure 7-37.
Figure 7-44 (right) Optic nerve atrophy is present in the glaucomatous left eye of the horse in Figure 7-37.

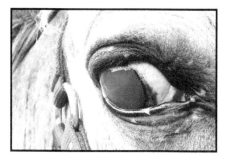
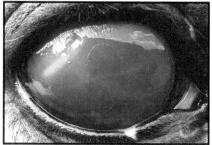

Figure 7-45 (left) Generalized corneal edema in a horse with glaucoma.

Figure 7-46 (right) Closeup of the eye in Figure 7-45. A few linear striate are present but difficult to see due to the edema.

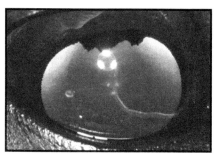
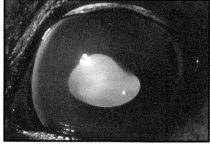

Figure 7-47 (left) Linear, thin areas of Descemet's membrane in a horse eye with normal IOP.

Figure 7-48 (right) Corneal edema and cataract in an old Thoroughbred mare with glaucoma. IOP was 80 mm Hg.

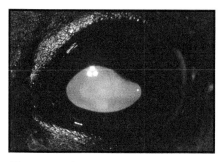
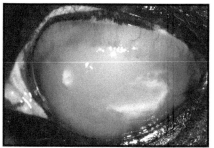

Figure 7-49 (left) The cornea is more clear and IOP reduced following transcleral cyclophotocoagulation in the eye in Figure 7-48. Buphthalmia occurred two years later.

Figure 7-50 (right) Corneal edema is so severe that an ulcer occurred in this horse with glaucoma.

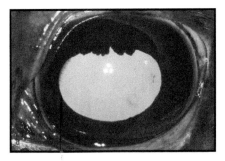 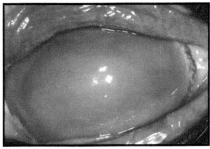

Figure 7-51 (left) Mydriasis in a Thoroughbred mare with glaucoma.
Figure 7-52 (right) Acute glaucoma produced severe corneal edema.

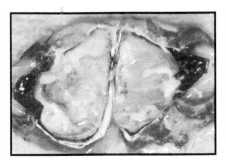 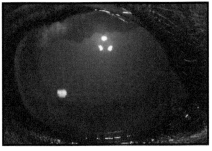

Figure 7-53 (left) Gross photograph of the globe in Figure 7-52 reveals extensive septic endophthalmitis from a gram negative bacterial infection.
Figure 7-54 (right) Generalized corneal edema and mydriasis in a Paso Fino stallion with glaucoma.

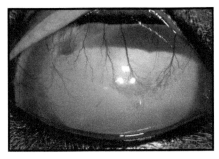 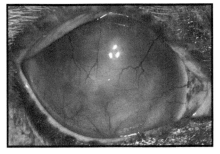

Figure 7-55 (left) The cornea has cleared and IOP diminished six months following transcleral cyclophotocoagulation in the eye in Figure 7-54.
Figure 7-56 (right) Chronic glaucoma has caused corneal edema and granulation tissue in this glaucomatous horse globe.

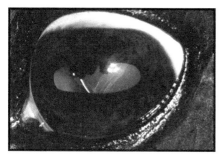

Figure 7-57 Lens luxation and large band opacity in a horse globe with glaucoma.

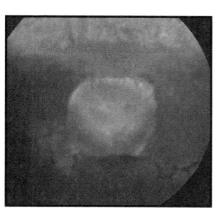

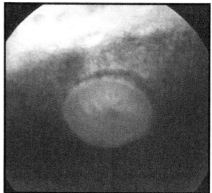

Figure 7-58 (left) Optic nerve atrophy and retinal scarring near the disc in an eye with glaucoma.

Figure 7-59 (right) Optic nerve cupping, disc pallor, and exposure of the scleral lamina cribrosa in a horse with chronic glaucoma.

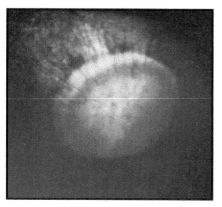

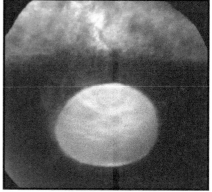

Figure 7-60 (left) The normal optic nerve in the other eye of the horse in Figure 7-59.

Figure 7-61 (right) Pale optic nerve and laminar exposure in a glaucomatous horse eye.

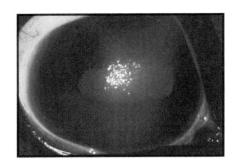

Figure 7-62 Vertical corneal edema is a precursor to glaucoma.

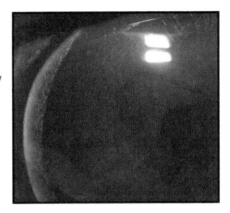

Figure 7-63 The grey line is the drainage angle in the horse. Brown pectinate ligaments attach to the grey line of the cornea and form the inner part of the drainage angle. Aqueous humor passes between the pectinate ligament and exits the eye here. A persistent pupillary membrane (PPM) is also present.

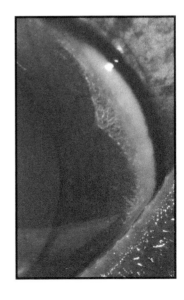

Figure 7-64 The angle has been distorted, focally stretched, and distended in an eye following trauma.

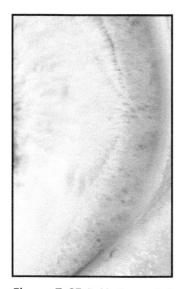 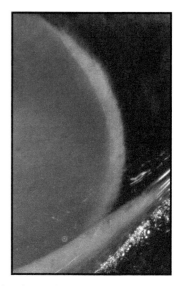

Figure 7-65 (left) The angle is white with red blood vessels visible in this subalbinotic horse eye.

Figure 7-66 (right) The angle is solid in appearance, and the drainage holes closed and collapsed in this horse eye with glaucoma.

☞ Vertical corneal edema in the central cornea may be an indicator of early glaucoma. This edema may arise from the convection currents found in the anterior chamber.

☞ The systemically administered carbonic anhydrase inhibitors acetazolamide (1-3 mg/kg QD, PO), the topical miotic pilocarpine (2.0% QID), the beta-blocker timolol maleate (0.5 % BID), and the topical carbonic anhydrase inhibitor dorzolamide (2.0% TID) have been utilized to lower IOP in horses with varying degrees of success. The newer prostaglandin derivatives cause low grade uveitis and may exacerbate the IOP in horses with glaucoma.

✓ Topical atropine therapy was once thought to reduce the incidence of glaucoma in horses with uveitis, but should be used cautiously with rigorous IOP monitoring in horses with glaucoma as it may cause IOP spikes.

✓ Anti-inflammatory therapy, consisting of topically and systemically administered corticosteroids, and/or topically and systemically administered nonsteroidal antiinflammatories also appear to be beneficial in the control of IOP.

☞ Laser destruction of the ciliary body (cyclophotocoagulation) works the best at controlling IOP and preserving vision in horses (see Figures 7-49, 7-55) and (Figure 7-67).

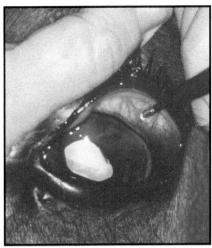

Figure 7-67 The eye in Figure 7-48 is receiving laser cyclophotocoagulation therapy for chronic glaucoma. The IOP remained stable for two years post-laser.

Contraindications/Possible Interactions

✓ Conventional glaucoma treatment with miotics such as the prostanglandindoids may provide varying amounts of IOP reduction in horses.

✓ Miotics and prostaglandins can potentiate the clinical signs of uveitis and should be used cautiously in horses with anterior uveitis.

8→ The horse eye seems to tolerate elevations in IOP for many months to years that would blind a dog, however, blindness is the end result.

✓ Buphthalmia can be associated with exposure keratitis.

✓ Topical atropine does not appear to have the benefit of lowering IOP in a majority of glaucomatous horse eyes as originally proposed.

Tips on Tonometry for Evaluation of Intraocular Pressure (IOP) in Horses

(courtesy of Dr Phil Pickett)

8→ 1. Topical anesthetic will make for the most reliable readings.

8→ 2. Minimal restraint, try not to excite the patient or IOPs will usually be artificially high.

👆 3. The Tono-Pen applanation tonometer is the most accurate tonometer available for horses.

👆 4. Do not push too hard on the cornea; one should not see the cornea indent when the tip touches it unless the IOP is very low.

👆 5. Make sure the tip comes into contact flat on the cornea, not at an angle; even a slight angle will reduce consistency of readings.

👆 6. Do not exert any pressure on the globe (i.e. forcibly prying open the lids will give erroneously high IOPs). Use the auriculopalpebral nerve block prior to IOP measurement.

👆 7. The tip cover should not be on too tight or too loose. The cover should be flat across the applanating tip, but there should be a little bit of wrinkling of the cover from the tip back. Too loose (where the cover is not in good contact with the instrument tip) can be very problematic, but I find that most people tend to put the cover on too tight. It can be very hard to get consistent readings (or any reading at all sometimes) if this is the case.

👆 8. Ophthalmic ointment on the cornea will cause erroneously high IOPs.

✓ 9. Watch the video and read the manual that comes with the instrument. Very self-explanatory.

The Uveal Tract

Heterochromia Iridis

✓ Heterochromia iridis, or dual coloration of the iris (usually blue and brown), is common to the Appaloosa, palomino, chestnut, gray, spotted, and white horses, and is not considered a true pathologic condition (Figures 7-68 to 7-70).

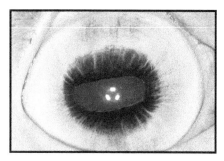 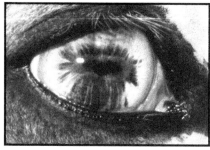

Figure 7-68 (left) Iris hypoplasia in a white horse.
Figure 7-69 (right) Iris hypoplasia and congenital miosis in a Paint horse.

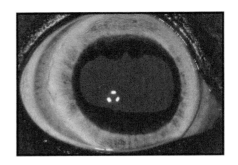

Figure 7-70 Normal heterochromic iris.

Aniridia/Iris Hypoplasia/Enlarged Corpora Nigra/Iris Colobomas

☞ Aniridia, or the complete absence of the iris, is reported in Quarter Horses and Belgians and is also seen with congenital cataracts in Thoroughbreds. Congenital thinning of the iris (hypoplasia) to a full thickness hole in the iris (coloboma) may be noted in heterochromic eyes (Figures 7-71 and 7-72). Enlargement of the corpora nigra can obstruct the pupil to cause vision problems.

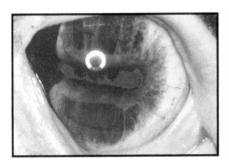
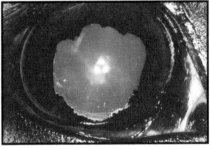

Figure 7-71 (left) The iris stroma is so thin and hypoplastic that the ventral equatorial rim of the lens can be seen.

Figure 7-72 (right) Congenital iris coloboma in a foal.

Iris and Ciliary Body Cysts

☞ ⊙ Uveal cysts are a hallmark of the hereditary anterior segment dysgenesis abnormalities of the Rocky Mountain Horse and the Connemara pony (Figures 7-73 to 7-76). Uveal cysts may be found sporadically in other breeds. Cysts of the iris, ciliary body and corporan nigra may occur. They are round and smooth and do not invade the iris as do their primary differential diagnosis the iris melanoma. The cysts contain a thick vitreous gel-like material.

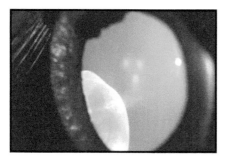
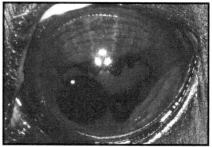

Figure 7-73 (left) Large ciliary cyst is seen posterior to the pupil in a Rocky Mountain horse with anterior segment dysgenesis.

Figure 7-74 (right) Iris cyst in a quarter horse that caused him to shy in certain situations.

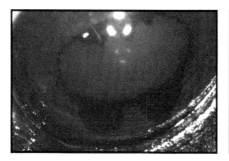
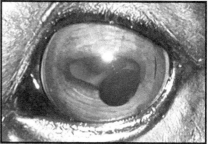

Figure 7-75 (left) Argon laser was used to collapse the cysts in Figure 7-74.

Figure 7-76 (right) Large iris cyst in a horse.

Cysts at the ventral pupil margin appear to cause more vision problems such as erratic behavior and head shaking. Iris cysts may become so large that they touch the corneal endothelium to cause ulcers. Cysts may be broken down with a laser or punctured with a needle (Video 26).

Equine Recurrent Uveitis (Periodic Ophthalmia, Moon Blindness, Iridocyclitis

✓ **Equine recurrent uveitis (ERU)** is a common cause of blindness in horses. It is a group of infectious and immune-mediated diseases of multiple etiologies.

✓ Recurrence or persistence of anterior uveitis is the hallmark of ERU. One to eight percent of the horses in the USA may have mild to severe ERU. In 2005 there were 9.2 million horses in the USA suggesting that there could be 736,000 cases!!

✓ The disease is bilateral in approximately 20% of the non Appaloosa cases, and 80% of the Appaloosas with ERU.

☞ Appaloosas are 8 times more likely to be affected by ERU than other horse breeds. Standardbreds are more resistant to developing ERU.

☞ Some Appaloosas appear to be "programmed" to develop ERU, as spotted Appaloosas are more likely than Appaloosas with lots of coat pigmentation to be affected. Brown eyes are more likely to be affected than heterochromic or blue eyes.

✓ German warmbloods positive to the leucocyte antigen ELA-A9 may have a heritable form of ERU.

☞ Appaloosas are genetically predisposed. The UM011 microsatellite had greater 182 allele in Appaloosas with ERU. The EqMHC1 microsatellite had greater 206 allele in Appaloosas with ERU.

☞ While the pathogenesis is clearly immune-mediated, the specific causes of ERU are unknown. Hypersensitivity to infectious agents such as *Leptospira interrogans* serovars is commonly implicated as a possible cause. Autoimmune activity against retinal proteins and antigens is also an etiologic component of this disease.

✓ The presence of living Leptospira organisms is not necessary for disease production, but has been found in the aqueous humor and vitreous of affected horses.

✓ Toxoplasmosis, brucellosis, salmonellosis, *Streptococcus, Escherichia coli, Rhodococcus equi*, borreliosis, intestinal strongyles, onchocerciasis, parasites such as *Halicephalobus deletrix*, and viral infections (e.g., equine influenza virus, herpes virus 1 and 4, arteritis virus, and infectious anemia virus) have also been implicated as causes of ERU with no consistency in isolation of these organisms from affected horses.

☞ Dead or dying microfilaria of *Onchocerca cervicalis* may release antigens to incite ERU following vascular migration to the eye of living microfilaria. Onchocerca treatment may incite uveitic attacks in horses with ERU.

✓ Deworming with ivermectin is associated with flareups of ERU in the USA.

✓ Anectodal cases of ERU occur 2-4 weeks following vaccination with various equine vaccines are reported.

✓ Leptospira infections in horses occur with exposure to urine or urine contaminated feed or water. Horses with insufficient vaccination or parasite prevention are more prone for viral and parasitic infections. The clinical signs of acute Leptospira infections are generally rather benign and self limiting, although inappetence, fever, icterus or abortions may be seen.

☞ Serologic testing for leptospirosis, brucellosis, and toxoplasmosis should be performed, although the results of serology can be difficult to interpret as many horses have positive titers with no evidence of ocular or systemic diseases. Not all horses positive for Leptospira have uveitis.

☞ Leptospiral titers for *L. pomona*, *L. bratislava* and *L. autumnalis* should be requested in the United States. Positive titers for serovars of 1:400 or greater are of importance.

♥ Serology for *Leptospira pomona* can be used for prognostic evaluation of the likelihood of blindness occurring in one or both eyes. Seropositive Appaloosas (100%) > seronegative Appaloosas (72%) > seropositive non-Appaloosas (51%) > serongegative non-Appaloosas (34%) at having blindness occur in at least one eye within 11 years of the first attack. Serologically positive horses to Leptospirosis have more aggressive clinical signs of disease.

✋ There are acutely active, and chronic quiet stages of ERU. The owner may think all is well in the quiescent eyes as the clinical signs are very subtle.

☞ Horses with ERU may display increased lacrimation, blepharospasm, and photophobia. Some horses with severe uveitis show no clinical evidence of pain!

☞ Subtle amounts of corneal edema, conjunctival hyperemia, and ciliary injection will be present initially, and can become prominent as the condition progresses. The edema may be only vertical in early cases of ERU, and more generalized later (see Figures 2-66 to 2-69) and (Figures 7-77 to 7-85).

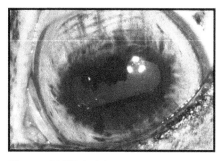 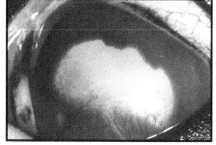

Figure 7-77 (left) Iris color change from ERU in an Appaloosa.

Figure 7-78 (right) Keratic precipitates (KPs) are leukocytes attached to the endothelium and appear as multiple dark spots in this eye with ERU.

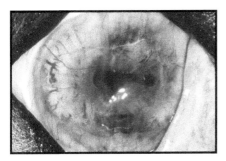
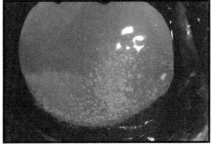

Figure 7-79 (left) Severe and persistent uveitis has caused iris color change, miosis, and iris vascularization in this 24 year old Appaloosa mare.

Figure 7-80 (right) Several white and a few brown keratic precipitates are present in the center and ventral part of the cornea in this eye with low grade uveitis.

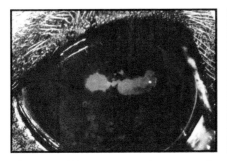
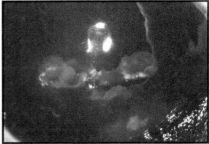

Figure 7-81 (left) Iris darkening and pupillary synechiation in a Lippazoner stallion with ERU (see Figures 3-21 and 3-22).

Figure 7-82 (right) Multiple corneal opacities in a horse with ERU. These became ulcerated eventually and developed band keratopathy.

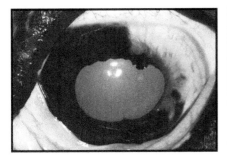
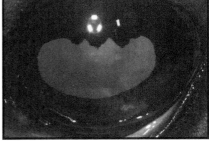

Figure 7-83 (left) Iris color change and vascularization of the iris in the blue area of this 24 year old Appaloosa caused by ERU.

Figure 7-84 (right) Cloudy vitreous in a horse with low grade ERU.

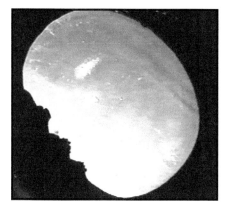

Figure 7-85 Small cataract in the horse in Figure 7-84 taken prior to cyclosporine A implant surgery.

✓ Aqueous flare, hyphema, intraocular fibrin, and hypopyon may be observed. Vitreal opacity occurs in some horses (see Figure 2-67) and (Figures 7-86 to 7-96).

☞ Miosis is usually a prominent sign and can result in a misshapen pupil and posterior synechiae. Delayed or failure to achieve pharmacologic mydriasis is common when uveitis is active. The corpora nigra atrophy in chronic ERU.

✓ A complete ophthalmic examination should be performed to determine if the uveitis is associated with a corneal ulcer. The presence of a corneal ulcer precludes the use of topical corticosteroids, but not topical nonsteroidal drugs.

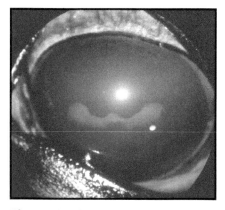
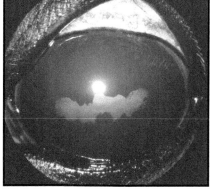

Figure 7-86 (left) Corneal edema, corneal vascularization, conjunctival hyperemia, and miosis are found in an eye with equine recurrent uveitis.

Figure 7-87 (right) Two days of medical therapy result in diminished corneal edema and conjunctival hyperemia. The pupil cannot dilate due to posterior synechia.

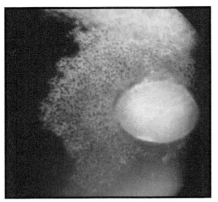
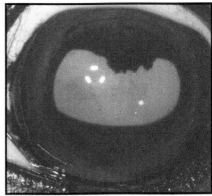

Figure 7-88 (left) Large area of retinal depigmentation to the left of the optic disc in a horse with equine recurrent uveitis.

Figure 7-89 (right) Vitreal haze and fibrin in an Appaloosa with acute equine recurrent uveitis.

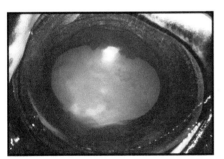
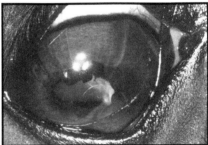

Figure 7-90 (left) Band keratopathy from chronic uveitis in a horse in England. (From Derek Knottenbelt).

Figure 7-91 (right) Small cataract due to a persistent pupillary membrane.

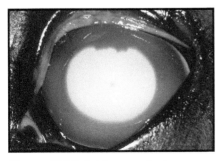
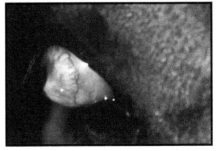

Figure 7-92 (left) Corneal edema caused by persistent uveitis in a warmblood gelding.

Figure 7-93 (right) Phthisical eye from persistent ERU.

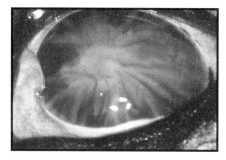 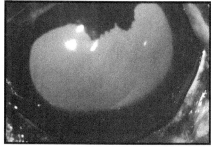

Figure 7-94 (left) The cornea is wrinkled due to hypotony in a phthisical eye with ERU.

Figure 7-95 (right) Vitreal yellowing in a warmblood with ERU.

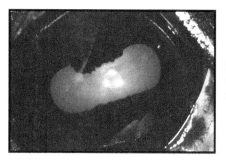

Figure 7-96 Cataract formation in the eye in Figure 7-95 occurred post-cyclosporine A implant surgery.

Intraocular pressure (IOP) is generally low, but ERU may be associated with intermittent and acute elevations in IOP. This "hypertensive uveitis" phase makes the diagnosis of glaucoma in horses difficult.

✓ Fibrin and iris pigment may be deposited on the anterior lens capsule.

✓ Cataract formation may occur rapidly if the inflammation does not subside quickly. Cataract formation is common to horses with with chronic ERU.

✓ Severe anterior segment inflammation often prevents an adequate fundic exam of the acutely affected eye (see Figures 2-66 to 2-69).

✓ Choroiditis may result in focal or diffuse retinitis, and exudative retinal detachments (see Figure 7-95).

✓ The vitreous may develop haziness due to leakage of proteins and cells from retinal vessels. Vitreal degeneration and liquefaction can occur (see Figure 7-89). Neutrophils cause the vitreous to have a greenish haze.

ϑ In chronic cases, corneal vascularization, permanent corneal edema, synechiation, band keratopathy, cataract formation, and iris depigmentation or hyperpigmentation can result. Secondary glaucoma and phthisis bulbi occur. Phthisical eyes may still have active uveitis and should be enucleated in many cases (see Figures 7-79, 7-82 to 7-94) and (Figures 7-97 to 7-99).

✓ ⊙ Retinal degeneration indicated by focal to generalized peripapillary regions of depigmentation in the nontapetum could result (see Figure 7-88) (Videos 31 to 34). The retinal degeneration may appear as linear bands of depigmentation in the nontapetal area.

✓ Solitary "bullet-hole" lesions cannot be used to make a diagnosis of ERU if no lesions of the anterior segment are present.

✓ The optic nerve head can appear congested.

✓ Inflammation of the pineal body is found in ERU.

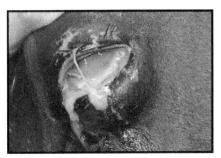 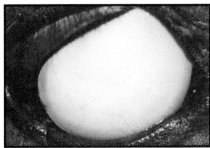

Figure 7-97 (left) Endophthalmitis and periorbital cellulilits secondary to accidental orbital formalin injection for ethmoid hematoma. (From Brian Burks).

Figure 7-98 (right) Complete bilateral corneal opacity secondary endophthalmitis due to septicemia from a penetrating foot injury. Right eye.

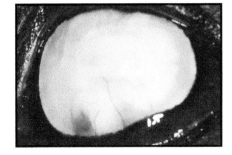

Figure 7-99 Corneal opacification in left eye in horse in Figure 7-98.

☞ Irreversible blindness is a common sequelae to ERU, and is due to retinal detachment, cataract formation or severe chorioretinitis.

☞ In acute stages, lymphocytic infiltration with some neutrophils can be found in the uveal tract, resulting in edema and plasmoid vitreous. T-lymphocytes are the predominant cell type. In addition, fibrin and leukocytes are present in the anterior chamber that manifests clinically as aqueous flare. Lymphocytes and plasma cells can surround the blood vessels of the iris, ciliary body, choroid, and retina. The chronic stages manifest corneal scarring, cataract formation, and peripapillary chorioretinitis with retinal degeneration and loss of photoreceptors. The retina and choroid are involved in all stages of ERU.

ERU Therapy

✓ The major goals of treatment of ERU are to preserve vision, decrease pain, and prevent or minimize the recurrence of attacks of uveitis. Specific prevention and therapy is often difficult, as the etiology is not identified in each case.

✓ Treatment should be aggressive and prompt in order to maintain the transparency of the ocular structures.

✓ Cataract surgery can be beneficial in the uveitic horse but does not cure the uveitis. Vision can be regained if the retina is healthy.

✓ Medications should be slowly reduced in frequency once clinical signs abate, but should continue at least 30 days past resolution of clinical signs.

✓ Therapy can last for weeks or months and should not be stopped abruptly or recurrence may occur.

Some Horses require Life-Long Therapy!

♥ Overall, the prognosis for ERU is usually poor for a cure to preserve vision, but the disease can be controlled. The Appaloosa breed seems to suffer from the most severe cases.

☀ It is imperative to immediately differentiate a painful eye in a horse as a result of ulcerative keratitis or stromal abscessation from the pain associated with ERU by employing a fluorescein dye test. While corticosteroids are the treatment of choice for ERU, they

can lead to the rapid demise of an eye with a corneal ulcer or abscess.

✓ The owner should be educated immediately about the potential recurrence, the blinding nature of this disease, and the possibility of enucleation to remove a painful eye if vision is lost. Annual vaccinations should be administered carefully in ERU horses.

☞ Anti-inflammatory medications, specifically corticosteroids and nonsteroidal drugs, are used to control the generally intense intraocular inflammation that can lead to blindness. Medication can be administered topically as solutions or ointments, subconjunctivally, orally, intramuscularly, and/or intravenously.

☞ Prednisolone acetate or dexamethasone should be applied initially.

✓ When the frequent application of topical steroids is not practical, the use of subconjunctival corticosteroids may be used. Systemic corticosteroids may be beneficial in severe, refractory cases of ERU, but pose some risk of inducing laminitis and should be used with caution.

☞ The nonsteroidal anti-inflammatory drugs (NSAID) can provide additive anti-inflammatory effects to the corticosteroids, and are effective at reducing the intraocular inflammation when a corneal ulcer is present. Cyclosporine A, an immunosuppressive drug, can be effective topically for ERU.

✓ Flunixin meglumine, phenylbutazone, or aspirin are frequently used systemically to control intraocular inflammation. Some horses become refractory to the beneficial effects of these medications, and it may be necessary to switch to one of the other NSAID to ameliorate the clinical signs of ERU.

✓ Topical atropine minimizes synechiae formation by inducing mydriasis, and alleviates some of the pain of ERU by relieving spasm of ciliary body muscles. It also narrows the capillary interendothelial cell junctions to reduce capillary plasma leakage.

✓ Although topically administered atropine can last 14 or more days in the normal equine eye, its effect may be only a few hours in duration in the inflamed ERU eye.

✓ The ease with which mydriasis can be achieved with intermittent use of atropine is an important indication as to the stimulus intensity of the ERU.

✓ Failure to achieve mydriasis with atropine indicates the stimulus for the ERU is quite prominent, and/or indicates the presence of synechiation.

☞ Observation of signs of abdominal pain and careful monitoring of gastrointestinal motility by abdominal auscultation is important when using topically administered atropine in horses and foals, as gut motility can be markedly reduced by atropine in some horses. Should gut motility decrease during treatment with topically administered atropine, one can either discontinue the drug or change to the shorter acting mydriatic tropicamide.

✔ The use systemically of topically administered antibiotics is often recommended for ERU. Antibiotics should be broad spectrum, and appropriate for the geographic location of the patient. Topical antibiotics are indicated in cases of uveitis due to penetrating ocular trauma, or ulcerative keratitis.

✔ Antibiotic treatment for horses with positive titers for Leptospira remains speculative but streptomycin (11 mg/kg IM BID) may be a good choice for horses at acute and chronic stages of the disease. Penicillin G sodium (10,000 U/kg IV or IM QID), enrofloxacin (7.5 mg/kg IV q24hr), and tetracycline (6.6 - 11 mg/kg IV BID) at high dosages may be beneficial during acute leptospiral infections. Treatment for leptospirosis does not appear to affect the outcome of ERU.

✔ Intravitreal gentamicin (4 mg/0.1ml) can benefit some horses with ERU.

☞ Tissue plasminogen activator (TPA) has been used to accelerate fibrinolysis and clear hypopyon in the anterior chamber of horses with severe iridocyclitis. An intracameral injection of 50-150 microg/eye can be made at the limbus with a 27-gauge needle under general anesthesia. TPA should be avoided if recent hemorrhage (< 48h) is present.

☞ Multivalent bovine and porcine leptospiral vaccines have been used in horses to treat intractable cases of ERU and to suppress herd outbreaks of leptospiral ERU, but their routine use as a preventative for ERU is controversial. Vaccination is best done in serologically leptospiral negative horses, but has been beneficial in some horses that were serologically positive. Vaccination with the porcine leptospiral vaccine reduced the recurrence of clinical signs of ERU from 57 to 35% in one study. It may have caused other horses to act "positive" so should be used with caution.

Alternative Therapy for ERU

✓ **Homeopathic remedies** (eg, poultices of chamomile and oral methylsulfonylmethane) for ERU have been used.

✓ **Acupuncture** has been used to treat ERU. All of the following acupoints can be used once every three days for treatment of active ERU: ST1 (stomach meridian # 1), GB1 (gall bladder meridian # 1), BL1 (bladder meridian # 1), and Jing-shu (Eye association point).

✓ **Phlebotomy** of Tai-Yang hemoacupuncture point (classical point #15) at the ipsilateral transverse facial vein 3cm caudal to the lateral canthus has anecdotal benefits in some acutely and chronically affected ERU eyes.

✓ **Cold laser therapy** is not recommended.

✓ **Green wavelength light phototherapy** can decrease inflammation in some ERU eyes.

✓ Historically, **"firing"** of the normal eye with caustic compounds was used to treat ERU of the affected contralateral eye, but cannot be recommended by me.

Surgical considerations for ERU

✓ In addition to medical treatment, **pars plana vitrectomy** in horses with ERU has been used successfully to remove fibrin, inflammatory cells and debris trapped in the vitreous leptospiral positive horses in order to improve vision and delay the progression of the clinical signs (see Figure 7-89) and (Figures 7-100 to 7-102). Vitrectomy is most beneficial in leptospiral positive horses with rather minor signs of uveitis, and horses with primarily vitreal changes.

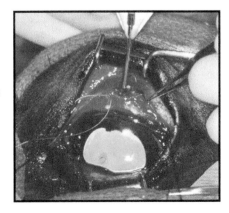

Figure 7-100 Pars plana vitrectomy is used for surgical therapy of equine recurrent uveitis.

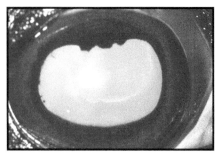
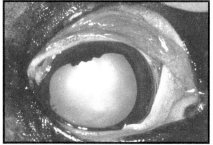

Figure 7-101 (left) Less haze and a vitreal cavity are found the day after pars plana vitrectomy in the horse in Figure 7-89.

Figure 7-102 (right) A mature cataract is found 2 months post-vitrectomy in the horse in Figure 7-89.

✓ ⊙ **Vitrectomy** appears more beneficial in European warmbloods with ERU than in Appaloosas and Quarter Horses with ERU in the USA. The reasons for this are not known. Cataracts occur in a high percentage of cases post-vitrectomy in both geographic regions. Retinal detachment can also occur postoperatively (Video 14).

⌇⊸ ⊙ Sustained release **intravitreal or subconjunctival cyclosporine A implants** may also be beneficial to treating ERU. Controlling the clinical signs medically is critical prior to implantation. CSA implants reduce the frequency and severity of uveitic attacks (Figures 7-103 to 7-107) (Video 13).

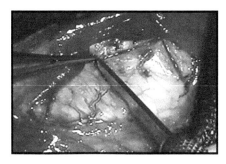
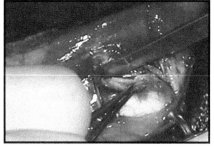

Figure 7-103 (left) The conjunctiva is incised and 3 scleral incisions made at the dorsal position to insert a cyclosporine A implant for horse in Figure 7-95.

Figure 7-104 (right) The sclera is very thick in the eye in Figure 7-95.

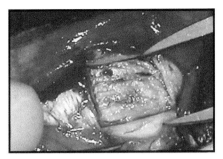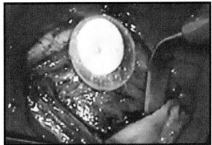

Figure 7-105 (left) The choroid is exposed under the scleral flap in the eye in Figure 7-95.

Figure 7-106 (right) The cyclosporine A implant is placed in the pocket created by the scleral incisions in the eye in Figure 7-95.

Figure 7-107 The sclera and conjunctiva are sutured in the eye in Figure 7-95.

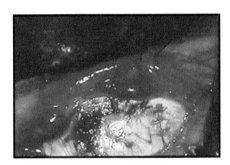

Section 8

Retinopathies and Ocular Manifestations of Systemic Diseases in the Horse

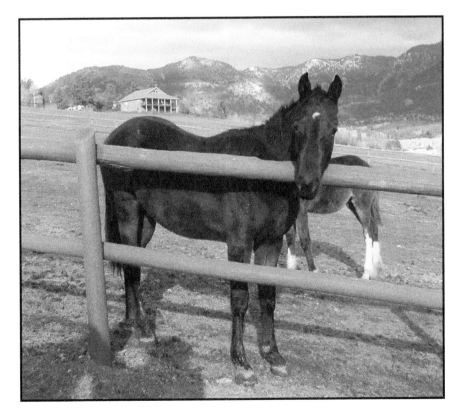

Retinopathies

Chorioretinitis

✓ ⊙ Chorioretinitis is inflammation of the choroid and retina. Inactive lesions are more often reported than active lesions. The tapetal region is rarely affected (Figures 8-1 to 8-9) (Videos 31 to 34).

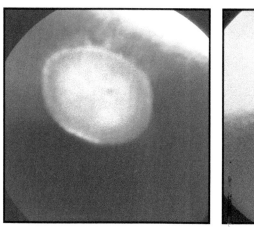
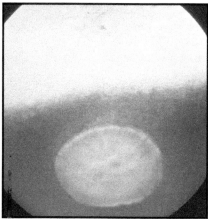

Figure 8-1 (left) Normal optic disc in a horse.
Figure 8-2 (right) Normal optic disc in a horse.

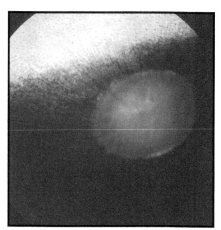
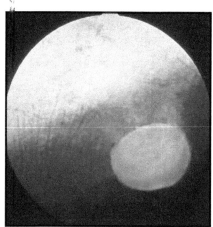

Figure 8-3 (left) The dark spots in the tapetum are normal capillaries penetrating the tapetum and are known as the Stars of Winslow.
Figure 8-4 (right) Choroidal vessels are noted in a horse with little retinal pigmentation.

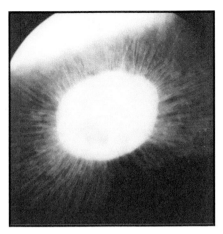 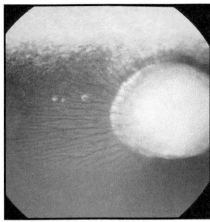

Figure 8-5 (left) Fluorescein angiography of a normal horse indicates the size of the retinal vessels, and their absence at the ventral edge of the optic disc.

Figure 8-6 (right) Several focal "bullet hole" chorioretinitis lesions manifest as focal areas of depigmentation with a hyperpigmented center. These spots are not associated with ERU.

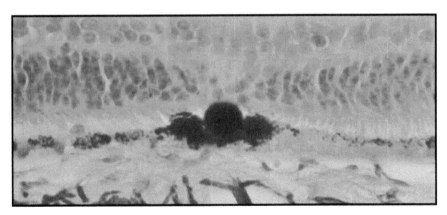

Figure 8-7 Histology of a focal chorioretinitis lesion noted in Figure 8-6 with an area of increased pigmentation of the retinal epithelium surrounded by a less pigmented area.

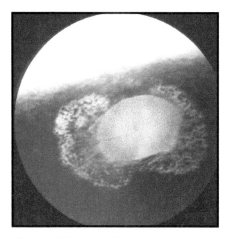 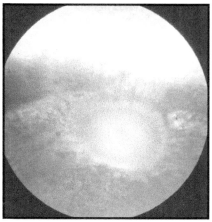

Figure 8-8 (left) Chorioretinal scarring near the optic disc in a horse with equine recurrent uveitis.

Figure 8-9 (right) Severe chorioretinal degeneration near the optic disc in a horse with equine recurrent uveitis.

⊶ It is manifested in equine eyes as focal "bullet-hole" retinal lesions, diffuse chorioretinal degenerative lesions, horizontal band lesions of the nontapetal retina, and chorioretinal degeneration near the optic nerve head. Multiple "bullet-hole" chorioretinal lesions can affect vision.

✓ Active chorioretinitis appears as focal white spots with indistinct edges, and as large diffuse gelatinous grey regions of retinal edema. Inactive chorioretinitis can appear as circular depigmented regions with hyperpigmented centers, or large areas of depigmentation that appear in some cases as the wings of a butterfly.

✓ Lesions can be caused by infectious agents (e.g., leptospirosis, EHV-1, EHV-4, *Onchocerca cervicalis*, *Rhodococcus*, *Streptococcus equi*, Lyme's disease, brucellosis, *Toxoplasmosis*, *Halicephalobus gingivalis*), immune-mediated uveitis of unknown origin, trauma, or vascular disease.

✓ Chorioretinitis may be found with or without the signs of anterior uveitis found with ERU.

✓ Serologic testing may identify infectious causes of chorioretinitis.

✓ Systemic NSAID medication is administered for chorioretinitis. Flunixin meglumine, phenylbutazone, or aspirin are indicated.

✓ Topical medication does not reach the retina and is only indicated if signs of anterior uveitis are also present.

Congenital Stationary Night Blindness

⊱┯ Congenital Stationary Night Blindness (CSNB) is found mainly in the Appaloosa, and may be inherited as a sex-linked or recessive trait. Up to 25% of Appaloosas may be affected. Cases are also noted in Quarterhorses, Thoroughbreds, Paso Finos, and Standardbreds.

⊱┯ Clinical signs include visual impairment in dim light with generally normal vision in daylight, and behavioral uneasiness and unpredictability occurring at night. CSNB does not generally progress, hence its name, but cases of progression to vision difficulties in the daytime are noted.

✓ Ophthalmoscopic examination is normal.

✓ Diagnosis is by clinical signs, breed, and ERG with decreased scotopic b-wave amplitude and a large negative, monotonic a-wave.

✓ CSNB appears to be caused by functional abnormality of neurotransmission in the middle retina.

✓ There is no therapy for this condition but affected animals should not be bred.

Equine Motor Neuron Disease Retinopathy

✓ **Retinal pigment epithelial cell accumulation of ceroid lipufuscin is found associated with the neurodegenerative condition, Equine Motor Neuron Disease (EMND). Generalized weakness, muscle fasciculations, weight loss, and muscle atrophy characterize EMND.**

⊱┯ Ophthalmic lesions are found in 40% of affected horses. A mosaic pattern of dark to yellow brown pigmentation (lipofuscin) in the tapetum of affected horses is noticed associated with a horizontal band of pigmentation at the tapetal-nontapetal junction (Figure 8-10). The nontapetum can also be affected.

⊱┯ Consistent evidence of a plasma vitamin E deficiency (<1.799 µg/ml) in horses with EMND suggests that the RPE, retinal, and spinal lesions are a result of oxidative injury associated with a prolonged deficiency of nutritionally derived antioxidants.

✓ While visual deficits may not be consistently found, nyctalopia and ERGs with a 50% reduction in b-wave amplitude and normal appearing a-waves have been noted associated with EMND.

✓ Supplementation with 6,000 IU vitamin E per day in horses with EMND may stabilize the neurologic signs, but it is not known if this will affect the RPE and retinal changes.

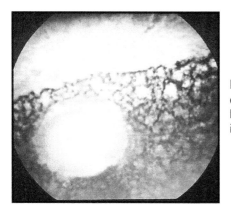

Figure 8-10 Equine motor neuron disease produces a mosaic pattern of hyperpigmentation and depigmentation in the nontapetum of this horse.

Retinal Detachments

✓ Retinal detachment is a separation of the nine layers of the sensory retina from the RPE. It is associated with slowly progressive or acute blindness in horses. It can be congenital in newborn foals or acquired later in life in adults.

✓ Retinal detachments can occur bilaterally or unilaterally, and be partial or complete.

✓ ⊙ Complete retinal detachments are seen clinically as free-floating, undulating, opaque veils in the vitreous overlying the optic disc. The tapetum is hyperreflective (Figures 8-11 and 8-12) (Videos 24 and 28).

♥ Retinal detachments are a complication of ERU, and are also associated with microphthalmos, head trauma, perforating globe wounds, cataract surgery, EPM, and may be secondary to tumors or vitreal degenerative processes. Retinal detachments can also be idiopathic. Chorioretinitis from EHV-1 and EHV-4 can result in giant retinal tears/detachments.

⌐ If the media of the eye are so opaque (e.g., corneal edema, cataract) that the fundus cannot be visualized, b-scan ultrasound can be used to diagnose the classic "seagull sign" of retinal detachment (Figure 8-13).

✓ Laser surgery and pneumatic retinopexy to reattach the retina are well described for the dog, but have not yet been reported for the horse.

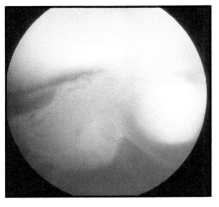 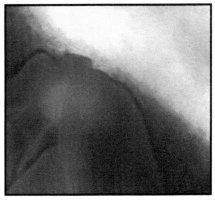

Figure 8-11 (left) Torn and folded retina obscures the optic disc in a retinal detachment in a foal.

Figure 8-12 (right) Retinal detachment following retinitis due to herpesvirous in a yearling.

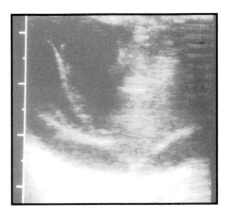

Figure 8-13 B-scan ultrasound reveals a cataract, retinal detachment and vitreal opacity in a horse with equine recurrent uveitis.

Optic Neuropathies

Optic Nerve Hypoplasia

✓ Congenital lack of retinal ganglion cell development, or excessive destruction of embryonic ganglion cells results in optic nerve hypoplasia. It may be unilateral or bilateral.

✓ Optic nerve hypoplasia may be associated with microphthalmos, cataracts, and retinal dysplasia.

✓ The optic discs are small and pale with fewer than normal retinal vessels present, and a one to four diopter posterior depression of the optic disc.

✓ Depending on the degree of optic nerve hypoplasia, slight visual impairment to total blindness may be noted.

✓ Mydriasis with slow to absent pupillary light reflexes (PLR) is present.

✓ There is no therapy for this nonprogressive condition.

Optic Nerve Atrophy

✓ Atrophy of the optic nerve can be due to inflammatory or noninflammatory causes.

✓ In the early stages the ophthalmoscopic appearance of the optic nerve head may be normal although the eye is blind. With time the optic disc becomes pale with profound vascular attenuation, and an obvious granularity of the optic disc due to exposure of the lamina cribrosa (Figure 8-14).

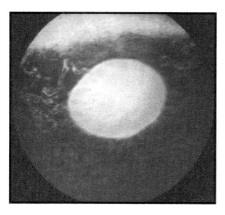

Figure 8-14 Optic nerve atrophy and blindness developed in a horse following head trauma.

✓ Blindness and pupil dilatation are the main clinical signs.

✓ Causes and risk factors include optic neuritis, equine recurrent uveitis, chorioretinitis, trauma, glaucoma, toxins, neoplasia, and bloodloss.

✓ Differential diagnosis includes optic nerve hypoplasia, retinal detachment, glaucoma, and cataract.

✓ There is no therapy for this condition.

Exudative Optic Neuritis

✓ This condition is found in older horses.

✓ Dilated pupils and sudden blindness occur in bilateral cases.

✓ ⊙ The optic discs in exudative optic neuritis are swollen with large whitish raised nodular masses spread across the surface of the optic disc. Retinal and optic disc hemorrhages may also be present (Video 25).

✓ The etiology is unknown.

✓ There is no known therapy and it has a poor prognosis for vision.

Proliferative Optic Neuropathy

✓ Proliferative optic neuropathy (PON) is primarly found in horses older than 15 years. It is generally unilateral with no signs of pain. There is little to no affect on vision in most cases and the PLRs are normal.

⌐ ⊙ A slowly enlarging white mass protruding from the optic disc into the vitreous can be noted ophthalmoscopically (Figure 8-15) (Video 35). The lesion is generally "fixed" and does not move when the eye moves. Some can be large enough to cast shadows on and stimulate the nearby retina.

✓ PON is a proliferation of granular cells from peripheral nerves that follow vessels into the optic disc. It resembles a Schwannoma histologically. Some may be extruded axoplasmic material rather than neoplastic.

✓ There is no therapy for this condition.

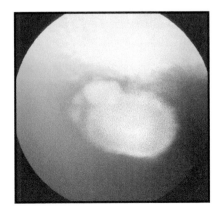

Figure 8-15 Mass at the dorsal margin of the optic disc is typical of proliferative optic neuropathy.

Ischemic Optic Neuropathy

✓ Head trauma, severe systemic hemorrhage, septic embolism, optic neuritis, and surgical ligation of the internal and external carotid and greater palatine arteries to eliminate epistaxis caused by guttural pouch mycosis are associated with ischemic optic neuropathy and sudden irreversible blindness in horses.

☞ Following sudden loss of blood supply, the optic disc at first appears slightly pale. Within 3 to 5 days white, raised lesions of the nerve fiber layer appear overlying the optic nerve and its margins. After several weeks there are ophthalmoscopic signs of retinal and optic nerve atrophy with pallor and vascular attenuation of the optic disc.

✓ Rapidly developing blindness, a dilated pupil, and absent PLR with no signs of pain are present.

✓ Treatment is symptomatic depending on the cause and whether any specific etiological agent has been identified.

✓ There is a very poor prognosis for return of vision.

Traumatic Optic Neuropathy

✓ Sudden blindness as a result of a horse falling over backwards and traumatizing its occipital crest can occur.

✓ Optic neuropathy results from tearing of the dural covering of the optic nerve, or direct compression of the optic nerve associated with hemorrhage or fractures of the basisphenoid bone.

☞ In early stages the optic disc may either appear normal, or edematous and hyperemic.

☞ There may be extrusion of optic disc axonal material into the vitreous. Rapid development of optic nerve atrophy is noted (see Figure 8-14).

☞ If bilateral, both pupils are dilated with no signs of eye pain.

✓ Immediate and aggressive systemic non-steroidal and/or steroidal antiinflammatory therapy may help preserve some vision.

Photic Headshaking

✓ Otherwise known as head tossing behavior, photic headshaking is a condition where, in the absence of any xternal stimuli other than light, a horse vigorously and violently shakes its head in horizontal, vertical, or rotary directions.

✓ This disorder is probably a form of optic-trigeminal nerve summation, where retina and optic nerve stimulation produces referred

216

sensation to the nasal cavity. The irritability in the nasal cavity causes the horse to shake its head.

✓ Hunter-type horses most commonly affected. Affected horses are 7 years old with mean duration of signs prior to referral of 8 months. Heritability is unknown. Geldings are over-represented.

✓ Excessive and occasionally violent rubbing, sneezing and flipping of the nose and head occur at rest or during exercise.

✓ Sunlight may stimulate parasympathetic activity in the infraorbital nerve resulting in irritating nasal sensations and headtossing. Most horses are asymptomatic in winter. Longer day length predisposes.

✓ Differential diagnoses for headshaking includeds otitis media/interna from mites, premxillary bone cysts, maxillary osteomas, guttural pouch disease, upper respiratory tract disease, bit and tack problems, and dental as well as ocular diseases such as iris cysts must also be ruled out as a cause.

✓ Radiography of skull and cervical spine to identify changes associated with otitis media and interna

✓ Blindfolding horse or placing in dark environments (improvement noted in headshakers), upper respiratory tract exam, endoscopy of the guttural pouches, tympanocentesis under general anesthesia (may be helpful to rule out ear disease that lacks radiologic evidence), thorough otic, oral, and ophthalmic exam, and bilateral infraorbital nerve blocks aid the diagnosis of photic headshaking.

✓ Headshaking can occur at rest or during exercise. Since most headshakers show signs shortly after the onset of activity, there may be unforseen risks in working an uncontrolled photic headshaker.

✓ Medical therapy controls, but does not cure the condition. If effective, medical treatment may only be needed during the season in which the horses exhibit headshaking behavior.

✓ If a horse does not respond to medical therapy and infraorbital nerve blocks are successful, the horse may be a candidate for bilateral infraorbital neurectomy.

✓ High dose, pulsed, oral dexamethose therapy has shown great promise in controlling this problem. 70 mg for 3 days in a row per month is recommended for three months, followed by 50 mg for 3 days for each month for a year. Half doses can be given later for maintenance.

✓ Cyproheptadine (H1 blocker), a serotonin antagonist which alters proopiomelanocortin (POMC) metabolism, has the potential to alleviate the clinical signs at a dose of 0.3 mg/kg PO BID for 7 days initially, then continued as needed. Some horses may require a dose up to 0.6 mg/kg PO BID. The antiepileptic drug carbamazepine can help others (10 mg/kg PO q6h, or 29 mg/kg PO q12h).

✓ A 7 day trial of cyproheptadine should determine whether the patient will respond favorably to medical management. Therapy can be stopped periodically and reinstated if the behavior recurs and there are no side effects.

✓ Horses kept in a dark environment may not show severe clinical headshaking. This type of management, however, may not be practical for the horse or its owner and trainer.

✓ A horse with uncontrolled headshaking may develop unwanted head trauma and the owner or trainer may find it difficult for the horse to optimally work or perform.

✓ Long term, seasonal medical therapy can control, but not cure this disease. Infraoribital nerve blocks relieved clinical signs in some horses. Posterior ethmoidal nerve (caudal nasal branch of the maxillary division of the trigeminal nerve) blocks were more effective in abolishing clinical signs. Neurectomies may eliminate headshaking signs indefinitely, but it should only be considered when medical therapy fails and temporary nerve blocks work.

Sudden Blindness

✓ Acute blindness may be associated with head or ocular trauma, ERU, glaucoma, cataracts, intraocular hemorrhage, exudative optic neuritis, retinal detachment, or CNS disease. Ivermectin toxicosis can cause blindness in foals. Intracarotid xylazine administration can cause blindness.

♥ Acutely blind horses are extremely agitated, anxious and dangerous.

⚷ Horses recovering from anesthesia following enucleation of sighted eyes for SCC can be very confused and agitated in the postoperative period. Extreme care should be utilized and the animals approached cautiously on the blind surgical side until the horse adapts to its condition.

Horses can adapt amazingly well to blindness, whether unilateral or bilateral, if allowed to adjust to their new condition. Several internet websites are devoted to the care of blind horses and other blind animals.

Ocular Manifestations of Systemic Diseases

✓ Several systemic infectious diseases have ocular signs in the horse. The ophthalmic signs may precede the manifestation of the systemic disease.

Bacterial Infections

Actinomyces

✓ Ocular signs include optic neuritis and exophthalmos.

Bacterial Meningitis

♥ Corneal ulcers from facial nerve dysfunction in bacterial meningitis is reported. Nystagmus, sluggish PLR, and absent menace reflexes are also reported in horses with bacterial meningitis.

Brucella abortus, B. melitensis

♥ This organism can cause iridocyclitis. A four fold or greater increase between paired serum samples 2 wk apart suggests recent exposure.

Clostridium tetani

✓ Tetanus is a highly fatal, infectious disease caused by the toxin of *Clostridium tetani*. The disease causes muscular rigidity, hyperesthesia and convulsions in horses of all ages. Despite the ready availability of cheap and effective prophylaxis, tetanus continues to cause sporadic equine mortality throughout the world. The most common route of infection is by wound contamination with spores. Disease results when conditions within the contaminated wound favor spore germination, bacterial proliferation and elaboration of toxin. Neglected puncture wounds are especially dangerous, but any break in the skin or mucous membranes is a potential portal of entry for C *tetani*.

✓ Signs are due to the potent exotoxin tetanospasmin, which is produced locally and reaches the CNS hematogenously and by passage along peripheral nerves. The toxin localizes in the ventral horn of the gray matter of the spinal cord and brainstem, binding irreversibly to gangliosides within synaptic membranes. The main action of tetanospasmin is to block the release of inhibitory neurotransmitter. Therefore, reflexes normally inhibited by descending inhibitory motor tracts or by inhibitory interneurons (polysynaptic reflexes) are greatly facilitated, resulting in tetanic contractions of muscles after normal sensory stimulation.

The most prominent ocular sign in horses with tetanus is prolapse of the nictitans, which may make a flickering motion when the horse is stimulated ("flick of the haw" or "flashing"). Other signs are facial muscle spasms, anxious expressions, flared nostrils, and erect ears. The eye may be enophthalmic because of retractor bulbi muscle contraction.

Clostridium botulinum

The exotoxin produced by this gram-positive rod is one of the most potent neurotoxins known. It prevents release of acetylcholine at all peripheral cholinergic junctions. Most cases follow ingestion of contaminated feed. Botulism can cause upper eyelid ptosis, and mydriasis with sluggish PLRs.

Leptospira pomona, L grippotyphosa

✓ Acute iridocyclitis and equine recurrent uveitis may be initiated by *Leptospira* species and sustained by irregularities in control of the autoimmune system. Peripapillary depigmented lesions may occur with acute or subacute infections of the fundus.

Lyme's Disease

✓ *Borrelia burgdorferi* is a spirochete that may cause mild iritis to severe panuveitis in horses. The life cycle of this organism involves deer and mice.

Neonatal septicemias

♥ Infection of the foal to cause septicemia can occur through different routes, including the placenta in utero, the respiratory tract, the gastrointestinal tract, or the umbilical stump. Gram-negative organisms predominate (85% of all confirmed cases) with E. coli being, by far, the most common isolate followed by Klebsiella pneumoniae, Salmonella spp., Enterobacter spp. and more, recently, Pasteurella spp. As far as isolation of gram-positive organisms at the University of Florida, Streptococcus spp. appear stable, Actinobacillus spp. are declining, and Enterococcus spp. are increasing. The incidence of Streptococcal and Actinobacillus infections appears to be on the rise at other institutions. Iridocyclitis can be found with neonatal septicemia caused by E. coli, Klebsiella, Salmonella, Actinobacillus, Pseudomonas, Pasteurella, Streptococcus, Bacillus, Corynebacterium, and others.

Rhodococcus equi

✓ *Rhodococcus equi* is a gram-positive macrophage pathogen. Iridocyclitis may accompany subclinical Rhodococcus pneumonia and septicemia in foals. Severe eye infections can cause an endophthalmitis.

Salmonella spp

♥ Salmonella infection is one of the most important causes of enteric disease in horses. Fatal infections occur in foals and in older debilitated horses. Septicemic horses may have signs ranging from conjunctival and scleral hemorrhages to a severe fibrinous iridocyclitis. *Salmonella* have been recovered from the anterior chambers of affected horses. Fibrin clots clear with topical and systemic treatment.

Streptococcus equi (strangles)

☞ Equine strangles is a highly contagious purulent lymphadenitis of the upper respiratory tract caused by the gram-positive *Streptococcus equi subsp. equi* (*S. equi*). Dissemination may be hematogenous or via lymphatic vessels and results in abscesses in lymph nodes and other organs of the thorax and abdomen. The lack of efficacy of neutrophils in phagocytosing and killing S. equi is due to a combination of the hyaluronic acid capsule, antiphagocytic M-protein (SeM), and a leukocidal toxin released by the organism. Although the disease primarily involves the upper airways and associated lymph nodes, spread to other locations may occur. A mucopurulent conjunctivitis develops with naturally occurring streptococcal infections. Severe bilateral iridocyclitis may occur. Multifocal chorioretinitis, optic neuritis, retinal hemorrhage, and retinal detachment have also been observed in foals. Intracranial abscesses can cause loss of pupillary reflexes, unilateral or bilateral blindness, nystagmus, head tremors, and/or head tilt. Guttural pouch infection by *Streptococcus equi* may lead to facial nerve palsy or Horner's syndrome.

Viral Infections

Equine Infectious Anemia

✓ The EIA virus is closely related to FIV. Tabanid fly vector transmission is most common. In severe cases conjunctival pallor and smaller retinal vessels are evident; hemorrhages of the conjunctivae and fundi also may occur.

Equine Viral Arteritis

✓ Equine viral arteritis (EVA) is an RNA virus that causes a panvasculitis. It can cause abortion in pregnant mares, and serious respiratory and intestinal disease in foals. Conjunctivits may be associated with a mucopurulent discharge. More severely affected horses develop eyelid and conjunctival edema. Keratitis and photophobia also may be present.

EHV-1 (Equine Abortion Virus) and EHV-4 (Rhinopneumonitis)

✓ The equine herpesviruses are highly contagious, prevalent and performance-limiting. These viruses can be immunosuppressive. Equine herpesvirus -1 and -4 have been isolated from horses with bilateral conjunctivitis and respiratory signs. EHV-1 afflicted horses may also have neurologic disease and associated blindness, strabismus, ptosis, iridocyclitis, KCS, facial nerve paralysis, retinal hemorrhage, chorioretinitis, or optic neuritis.

EHV-2 (Equine Cytomegalovirus)

✓ EHV-2 has been found in corneal ulcers in horses in Florida. A unilateral keratoconjunctivitis with respiratory signs has been noticed in foals. EHV-2 may predispose to *Rhodococcus*.

Equine Viral Encephalitis (eastern (EEE), Western (WEE), and Venezuelan (VEE))

✓ These three viruses are infectious, zoonotic viruses of horses and humans. All of these viruses are maintained in nature by sylvatic cycles involving mosquito vectors and bird and other animal reservoirs. No case of VEE has been reported in the US since 1971, though a focus of enzootic VEE virus exists in the Everglades region of Florida without associated equine disease. Mortality ranges from 75% to 95% for EEE, 19% to 50% for WEE, and 40% to 90% for VEE.

✓ Ocular findings are blindness, nystagmus, facial paralysis, and exposure keratitis. Horses that survive may have permanent visual deficits. VEE is less common in the USA. An affected horse may stand in a stupor with its eyes closed and lip drooping, or it may walk and seem blind.

Adenovirus

✓ Adenoviruses are widely distributed in the horse population. Infection is rarely associated with disease in immunocompetent adult horses. Infection with adenovirus can be a problem in immunocompromised foals, especially Arabian foals with combined immunodeficiency syndrome. A mild to severe mucopurulent conjunctivitis may be present in foals infected with equine adenovirus. Giemsa- or H&E-stained conjunctival scrapings demonstrate deep reddish purple intranuclear inclusion bodies. The infection may cause a keratitis or a panuveitis.

Chlamydial Infections

✓ A keratoconjunctivitis may be the only disease produced with some chlamydial infections in horses.

Fungal Infections

Cryptococcus Neoformans

✓ Central nervous system involvement by this organism produces blindness. Optic nerve infections may cause an optic neuritis. Intraocular infections may produce a chorioretinitis or anterior uveitis. Nasal, sinus, and guttural pouch granulomas extend into the orbit and cause Horner's syndrome or a facial nerve palsy.

Histoplasma Farciminosus, H. Capsulatum (Epizootic Lymphangitis)

✓ These organisms cause a blepharitis and purulent conjunctivitis. Ulcerating wounds or cords of suppurative lymphangitis often occur below the eye. Although most granulomas are conjunctival, about 17% appear along the free margin of the lower eyelid.

Fungal Guttural Pouch Infection (Gutturomycosis)

✓ The facial nerve traverses the dorsolateral ceiling of the guttural pouch. The cranial sympathetic trunk, closely associated with the common carotid artery, may become involved in an inflammatory process of the pouch. There can be Horner's syndrome, facial nerve palsy, and/or blindness. Ipsilateral ptosis, photophobia, lacrimation, and miosis can occur. Blindness may be due to compression of the optic nerve or chiasm by a fungal granuloma, or it may follow an infarction. Endoscopy of the guttural pouch will help confirm the diagnosis.

Protozoan Infections

Toxoplasma Gondii

✓ Peripapillary chorioretinitis and optic nerve atrophy can occur in horses with toxoplasmosis. The organism may figure in the etiology of ERU.

Babesia sp

✓ Babesial infections are tick-borne hemoprotozoans that stimulate lacrimation. Edema of the eyelids and supraorbital fossae may be prominent. Petechiae and ecchymoses of the nictitans and conjunctiva occur. Blood may be present in the tears, and the conjunctiva may be icteric.

Equine Protozoal Myeloencephalitis (EPM)

♥ Equine protozoal myeloencephalitis (EPM) is a common neurological disease of horses in the Americas. A causative agent, Sarcocystis neurona, has been isolated from affected horses and serologic surveys suggest that up to 50% of horses in the US have been infected with this agent. The Virginia opossum is the definitive host. There is some evidence that the prevalence of the disease has dropped during the last 5 years. EPM is considered a treatable disease (TMS+pyrimethamine) although the response to therapy is often incomplete.

♥ Horses with EPM most commonly have abnormalities of gait but also may present with signs of brain disease. The disease ranges in severity from mild lameness to sudden recumbency and clinical signs usually are progressive. A variety of neurologic signs are possible as the organism can proliferate in any part of the CNS. Ophthalmic signs (blindness, nystagmus, ptosis, and head tilt) may be highly variable and nonspecific. Corneal anesthesia from a trigeminal neuropathy may be noticed. Cysts containing the parasites are found in the extraocular muscles.

Neoplasia

Lymphoma

✓ The initial clinical sign may be a uni- or bilateral anterior uveitis. The anterior chambers will contain blood, and the irides may be thickened and swollen. Other ocular lesions include masses on the nictitans, chemosis of the conjunctiva, and infiltration of the eyelids by neoplastic cells.

Pituitary Adenoma

♥ Because the pituitary in horses is below the tuber cinereum medially, and the optic tracts laterally, adenomas usually do not compromise the visual system directly. A distended third ventricle will push against the optic chiasm. They may, however, interfere with the blood supply to the optic pathways and thus indirectly produce blindness. A common manifestation of pituitary adenoma is a long shaggy coat.

Unknowns

Equine Mare Reproductive Loss Syndrome

♥ This group of diseases noted in Kentucky in 2001 consisted of horses affected in 3 distinct groups. There were yearlings with severe uveitis, mares with abortions, and other horses with pericarditis. The feces of caterpillar feeding from cherry trees contained cyanide and may have contributed to the pathogenesis. Systemic bacterial infection may also have been involved.

Eye Diseases associated with Specific Horse Breeds

Appaloosa

Congenital stationary night blindness

Congenital cataracts

Glaucoma

ERU

Optic disc colobomas

SCC

Arabian

Congenital cataracts

Vitiligo

Atropine sensitivity

Belgian draft horse

Aniridia and secondary cataracts

SCC

Morgan

Cataracts: nuclear, bilateral, symmetrical, and non-progressive

Quarter Horse

Congenital cataracts

Entropion

Thoroughbred

Congenital cataracts

Microphthalmia associated with multiple ocular defects

Retinal dysplasia associated with retinal detachments in some cases

Entropion

Color-Dilute Breeds

Iridal hypoplasia (photophobia)

SCC

Standardbred

Retinal detachments

Congenital stationary night blindness

Paso Fino

Congenital stationary night blindness

Glaucoma

American Saddlebred

Cataracts

Esotropia

Aggressive keratomycosis

Warm Bloods

Glaucoma

ERU

Rocky Mountain Horse (chocolate coat color most often affected)

Anterior segment dysgenesis: Collectively the cornea, iris and ciliary body lesions are termed anterior segment dysgenesis (ASD).

Congenital miosis, and corpora nigra and iris hypoplasia

Macrocornea

Ciliary Body Cysts (temporal)

Cataract, Lens Luxation

Retinal Dysplasia, Retinal Detachment

Miniature Horses

Upper lid entropion

Connemara Pony

Anterior segment dysgenesis

Mules

Aggressive sarcoid

Misplaced nasolacrimal puncta

Haflinger

SCC predisposed

Lippizzaners

Sarcoid resistant

Percherons

Melanomas

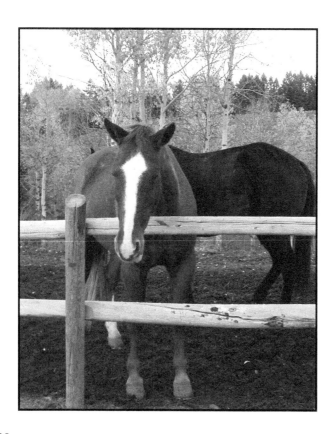

Links

Blind horse storey: www.valianttrust.org and sanctuary: www.blindhorses.org, http://www.blindappaloosas.org/index.html

American College of Veterinary Ophthalmologists: www.acvo.com

American Association of Equine Practitioners: www.aaep.org

European Society of Veterinary Ophthalmology: www.esvo.com

Electroretinography in Horses

Method 1: A method for the recording of flash electroretinograms (ERGs) in sedated, standing horses with the DTL™ microfiber electrode was developed. The pupil is dilated and the auriculopalpebral nerve blocked. The horse is sedated intravenously with detomidine hydrochloride (0.015 mg/kg). The sedation lasts 20-30 minutes. The ERGs are recorded with the active electrode on the cornea (DTL™), the reference electrode near the lateral canthus, and the ground electrode over the occipital bone. The light intensities of the white strobe light are 0.03 cd·s/m (scotopic) and 3 cd·s/m (scotopic and photopic). Photopic and scotopic single flash and flicker responses to Ganzfeld stimulation can be recorded. During the 20 minutes of dark adaptation period the retina is stimulated every 5 minutes with the 0.03 cd·s/m single flash.

The median b-wave amplitudes and implicit times were 38 µV and 33 ms (photopic cone-dominated response), 43 µV and 63 ms (5 minutes dark adaptation), 72 µV and 89 ms (10 minutes dark adaptation), 147 µV and 103 ms (15 minutes dark adaptation), 188 µV and 109 ms (20 minutes dark adaptation, 0.03 cd·s/m, rod response), and 186 µV and 77 ms (20 minutes dark adaptation, 3 cd·s/m , maximal combined rod-cone response). A steady increase in amplitude and implicit time was noted during dark adaptation. No oscillatory potentials could be isolated.

Method 2: The electroretinogram (ERG) of horses can be measured under xylazine sedation (0.5 mg/kg). Contact lens electrodes (#7506 ERG-Jet disposable contact lens electrode, The Electrode Store, Ehumclaw, WA; (800) 537-1093) are placed on the cornea (positive electrode), at the lateral canthus of the stimulated eye (negative electrode), and the ground electrode placed 1 cm from the crown of the head or vertex (Figure 2-21).

The mean latencies and amplitudes of the photopic a and b waves are 5.19 ± 1.56 and 26.63 ± 2.26 ms, and 40.89 ± 20.50 and 184.75 ± 63.26 µV, respectively.

The mean latencies and amplitudes of the low intensity flash (0.33 CDs/m2 with five minutes of dark adaptation) scotopic a- and b-waves are 5.73 ± 1.88 and 36.95 ± 3.89 ms, and 103.18 ± 120.72 and 409.30 ± 319.36 µV, respectively.

The mean latencies and amplitudes of the high intensity flash (4.62 CDs/m2 after five minutes of dark adaptation) scotopic a- and b-waves are 5.13 ± 1.34 and 34.75 ± 1.87 ms, and 153.68 ± 94.19 and 374.09 ± 161.93 µV, respectively.

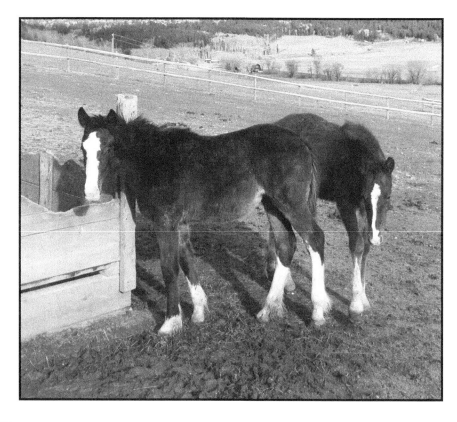

Lavage Treatment Systems

Horses with painful eyes may be difficult to treat with topical medications. Subpalpebral or nasolacrimal lavage treatment systems are employed for frequent treatment of fractious horses with painful eyes.

Various techniques have been described, although the method that I prefer utilizes silicone tubing with a single hole and foot-plate positioned in the superior palpebral fornix.

Sedation, eyelid akinesia, sensory eyelid blocks, and topical anesthesia are generally sufficient for placement of this tubing system.

Lavage tubing runs from the fornix to the withers. Medication is injected at the withers, runs through the tubing, exits at the footplate under the lid, and then flows over the corneal surface. Injections are spaced several minutes apart to prevent dilution of the medications.

Commercially available lavage kits (Mila Eye Lavage Kit) with a sterile 12-gauge hubless needle, and silicone tubing (0.065 inch OD) with a footplate attached at one end to prevent the tubing pulling out of the lid are very useful. 0.2 ml of drug are injected at each treatment period, the tubing is gently flushed with air, and the process then repeated for the next drug. Infusion pumps may be attached to the lavage systems to provide continuous perfusion of medications onto the cornea.

Address for MILA:
Email: www.milaint.com
MILA International, Inc.
7604 Dixie Hwy.
Florence, KY 41042 USA
FAX: 859-3714792
Phone: 859-371-172

Glossary of Selected Veterinary Ophthalmic Terms

Ophthalmic terminology is extensive and challenging to use!

Accommodation: the adjustment of the eye for seeing at different distances. In most animals, it is produced by a change in the shape of the lens, especially the anterior surface.

Adnexa: appendages of the eye (eyelids, conjunctiva, extraocular muscles, and glands of the orbit).

Aniridia: absence of the iris.

Anisocoria: difference in size of the pupils.

Anterior chamber (AC): space in the eye bounded in front by the cornea and behind by the iris and pupil; filled with aqueous humor.

Anterior segment: the anterior portion of the globe (cornea, iris, lens, anterior and posterior chamber, and anterior sclera).

Aphakia: absence of a lens.

Aqueous: aqueous humor; clear watery fluid that fills the anterior and posterior chambers of the eye.

Aqueous flare: visualization of a beam of light as it passes through the usually transparent aqueous of the anterior chamber; seen with an increase in protein as a result of uveitis.

Binocular vision: the ability to use the two eyes simultaneously to focus on the same object and to fuse the two images into a single image (depth perception).

Blepharitis: inflammation of the eyelids.

Blepharoplasty: eyelid surgery

Blepharospasm: sustained contraction of the orbicularis oculi muscle.

Buphthalmos: enlargement of the entire eye, as in glaucoma; hydrophthalmos and buphthalmia are synonyms.

Canthotomy: incision of the canthus to increase exposure of the globe for surgery.

Canthus: the anatomical region at either end of the eyelid aperture where the upper and lower eyelids adjoin; specified as lateral or temporal, and medial or nasal (pl. canthi).

Cataract: any opacity of the lens or its capsule or both.

Chemosis: edema of the conjunctiva.

Chorioretinitis: inflammation of the choroid and retina.

Choroid: the posterior uveal vascular region that furnishes nourishment to the retina.

Ciliary body: the portion of the uveal tract between the iris and the choroid; consists of ciliary processes and ciliary muscles.

Coloboma: a congenital fissure or cleft of any part of the eye or eyelid; commonly divided into typical (seen at 6 o'clock) and atypical colobomas.

Conjunctivitis: inflammation of the conjunctiva.

Corpora nigrum: (granula iridica) pigmented irregular mass on the dorsal and/or the ventral pupillary margin of the iris in herbivores.

Cyclitis: inflammation of the ciliary body.

Cyclocryotherapy: application of an ultra-cold probe on the sclera to freeze and destroy the ciliary body epithelium to reduce aqueous humor formation in the control of glaucoma.

Cyclophotoablation: the use of laser energy to destroy portions of the ciliary body in treatment of glaucoma.

Cycloplegia: paralysis of the ciliary muscle resulting in loss of accommodation.

Cycloplegic: a drug that temporarily paralyzes the ciliary muscle; pupillary dilatation also results due to iris sphincter paralysis. Atropine and tropicamide are examples.

Dacryocystitis: inflammation of the lacrimal sac and/or nasolacrimal duct.

Dacryocystorhinography: radiopaque study of the nasolacrimal system.

Dacryocystorhinostomy: surgical procedure to construct an alternate nasolacrimal drainage system.

Dermoid: a congenital growth (choristoma) consisting of skin and its dermal appendages. Usually located near or connected to the lateral canthus involving cornea, sclera, and conjunctiva.

Descemetocele: a deep corneal ulcer characterized by exposure and possible protrusion of Descemet's membrane.

Diopter: the unit in which the refracting strength of a lens is designated. One diopter (D) has a focal length of one meter and two diopters has a focal length of 0.5 meters.

Distichiasis: the presence of two separate rows of cilia on one eyelid; the abnormal cilia usually originate from the meibomian glands. Individual aberrant cilia are termed distichia.

Dyscoria: abnormal shape or reaction of the pupil

Ectopic cilia: cilium/cilia protruding through palpebral conjunctiva.

Ectropion: an eversion or turning out of the eyelid margin.

Ectropion uveae: eversion of the pigmented posterior iris tissue around the pupillary margin.

Electroretinography: (ERG), recording of retinal electrical potentials generated by flashes of light.

Endophthalmitis: inflammation of the inner layers of the eye.

Entropion: an inversion or turning inward of the eyelid margin.

Enucleation: removal of the globe leaving the extraocular muscles and other orbital tissues.

Epiphora: an overflow of tears onto the face.

Equine Recurrent Uveitis (ERU): recurrent iridocyclochoroiditis of horses. Lay terms = "moon blindness" and "periodic ophthalmia."

Esotropia: strabismus in which there is manifest deviation of the visual axis of an eye toward that of the other eye. Called also cross-eye and convergent or internal strabismus.

Evisceration: removal of the internal contents of the eye with retention of the fibrous coat (cornea and sclera).

Exenteration: removal of the eyeball and all soft tissues within the bony orbit.

Exophthalmos: protrusion of the eyeball from its normal position in the orbit.

Exotropia: strabismus in which there is permanent deviation of the visual axis of one eye away from that of the other. Called also divergent or external strabismus, and walleye.

Floaters: particles in the vitreous that can be of inflammatory or noninflammatory origin.

Fluorescein: water-soluble compound that yields a bright green fluorescence with cobalt blue illumination. Used for detection of corneal ulcers, and evaluation of the integrity of the blood-aqueous barrier and the patency of the nasolacrimal drainage apparatus.

Fornix: the junction of the palpebral and bulbar conjunctivas.

Fundus: the posterior layers of the eye that can be seen with an ophthalmoscope.

Glaucoma: abnormal increase in intraocular pressure (IOP) above that which is compatible with normal function of the eye.

Heterochromia: difference in color of the two irides, or two or more colors in the same iris.

Horner's syndrome: usually a unilateral disease resulting from sympathetic denervation; signs include protrusion of the nictitating membrane, ptosis, and miosis in most species.

Hyperopia: a refractive error in which the focal point of light rays from a distant object is behind the retina (farsightedness).

Hypertropia: vertical strabismus in which there is permanent downward deviation of the visual axis of an eye.

Hyphema: hemorrhage in the anterior chamber of the eye.

Hypopyon: inflammatory cells (neutrophils) in the anterior chamber.

Hypotony: abnormally low intraocular pressure.

Hypotropia: vertical strabismus in which there is permanent downward deviation of the visual axis of an eye.

Iridectomy: surgical excision of a portion of the iris.

Iridocyclitis: inflammation of the iris and ciliary body, also anterior uveitis.

Iridodonesis: trembling of the iris with movement of the eye, indicating loss of lens support.

Iridotomy: incision of the iris.

Iris bombé: posterior synechia that develop during uveitis block the outflow of aqueous humor into the anterior chamber, elevated posterior chamber pressure due to the accumulation of aqueous humor in the posterior chamber, and cause the iris to bow forward and result in a reduction in anterior chamber depth.

Iritis: inflammation of the iris, marked by miosis, aqueous flare and iris discoloration.

Keratic precipitates (KPs): inflammatory cell aggregates attached to the endothelial surface of the cornea; appear as multifocal white to dark opacities in the mid to ventral cornea in uveitis.

Keratitis: corneal inflammation. Can be ulcerative or nonulcerative.

Keratoconjunctivitis sicca: (KCS) dry cornea and conjunctiva, usually as a result of lacrimal gland deficiency.

Keratoplasty: corneal grafting, either partial thickness (lamellar) or full thickness (penetrating); may be done for therapeutic, tectonic or optical reasons.

Lagophthalmos: an inability to close the eyelids completely.

Lamina cribrosa: modified area of the sclera where optic nerve fibers pass from the globe.

Lenticonus: conical projection of the anterior or posterior surface of the lens.

Leukoma: a large diameter, dense, corneal opacity.

Limbus: boundary between the cornea and sclera.

Megalocornea: congenitally large cornea that may be confused with congenital glaucoma.

Meibomian glands: sebaceous gland in the eyelids with duct openings onto the eyelid margin.

Microphthalmos: an abnormally small eyeball.

Miosis: constriction of the pupil.

Miotic: a medication causing the pupil to constrict.

Mydriasis: dilation of the pupil.

Mydriatic: a medication causing the pupil to dilate.

Myopia: a refractive error in which the point of focus for rays of light from distant objects is in front of the retina (nearsightedness, myopic).

Nyctalopia: night blindness.

Nystagmus: an involuntary, rapid movement of the eyeball, either horizontal, rotary or vertical.

OD: abbreviation for right eye (oculus dexter, Latin).

OS: abbreviation for left eye (oculus sinister, Latin).

OU: abbreviation for both eyes (oculus uterque, Latin).

Optic axis: imaginary line from the center of the fundus through the center of the lens and cornea.

Optic disc: visible portion of the optic nerve in the fundus of the eye; also called the optic nerve head and optic papilla.

Panophthalmitis: inflammation involving all structures of the eye.

Papilla: the optic disc or optic nerve head.

Penetrating: a wound entering an ocular structure but not going completely through it.

Perforating: a wound completely traversing an ocular structure.

Photophobia: abnormal sensitivity to and discomfort from light.

Phthisis bulbi: shrunken and atrophic globe.

Plasmoid aqueous: fibrin in the anterior chamber, abnormal increase in protein in the anterior chamber.

Posterior segment: portion of the eye posterior to the lens that includes the vitreous, retina, choroid, and optic nerve.

Proptosis: forward protrusion or luxation of the eyeball, usually resulting from trauma.

Ptosis: drooping of the upper eyelid.

Pupil: the opening in the center of the iris.

Refraction: deviation in the course of light rays passing from one transparent medium into another of different density; determination of refractive error of the eye and correction by various lenses.

Retroillumination: to illuminate from behind by reflecting light from a deeper structure; eg reflect light off the tapetum to examine the lens.

Rose bengal: topical ophthalmic stain used to detect dead, degenerating, and devitalized corneal and conjunctival cells, and mucin tear layer defects.

Schirmer Tear test: method of measuring tear production using filter paper.

Sclerectomy: excision of a portion of the sclera.

Sclerotomy: incision of the sclera.

Seidel's test: aqueous humor leaking through a corneal perforation alters the color of fluorescein dye placed on the cornea.

Strabismus: The visual axes assume a position relative to each other different from that required by the physiological conditions. The deviation of the eyes is such that binocular fixation is impossible.

Stars of Winslow: end on view of small vessels penetrating the tapetum to connect deeper choroid vessels to the choriocapillaris; seen as a mosaic of regularly spaced minute dark foci (prominent in herbivores).

Striate Keratopathy: irregular linear opacities in the cornea usually associated with changes in Descemet's membrane. Seen in glaucoma (breaks in Descemet's) and phthisis bulbi (folding of Descemet's).

Symblepharon: adhesion of one or both eyelids to the globe.

Synechia: adhesion of the iris to cornea (anteriors.), or lens (posteriors.); plural, synechiae. It only takes seconds for synechia to form due to fibrin acting as tissue glue. Vascularization of synechia occurs with time.

Tapetum: reflective layer within the choroid that increases night vision capability.

Tarsorrhaphy: suturing together of the eyelids.

Tectonic: corneal grafting to replace damaged or lost cornea for structural rather than optical reasons.

Tenon's capsule: fibrous sheath enveloping most of scleral portion of the globe; episcleral fascia.

Thermatokeratoplasty: Focal disruption of the corneal epithelium with heat or cautery to allow fluid movement from the stroma to the tear film.

Tonometry: measure of intraocular pressure (IOP).

Transillumination: passing a light beam through a structure or tissue.

Trichiasis: normally placed but abnormally directed cilium.

Uvea: vascular layer of the eye that includes the iris, ciliary body and choroid. The anterior uvea consists of the iris and ciliary body, and the posterior uvea is the choroid.

Uveitis: inflammation of the uvea (vascular coat of the eye).

Visual acuity: Light waves emanating from objects in the visual field form miniaturized retinal images. The contour of each image is determined by the contrast produced between stimulated and unstimulated photoreceptors. The contrast sensation results in the perception of shape, size, and relative location of objects. The maximal perception of contour is known as best visual acuity.

Visual axis: imaginary line connecting a viewed object and the most sensitive area of the retina.

Visual field: the area that can be seen without shifting the gaze; can apply to that of both eyes or each eye separately.

Zonules: fine tissue ligaments that connect the lens to the ciliary body.

Treatment Plans/Practice Tips

I. Sarcoid Therapy

Intralesional cisplatin is administered in four or more sessions at two-week intervals using 1 mg/cm^3 of tumor. Tumors up to 20 cm^3 in size may be treated using 3.3mg/ml cisplatin (10 mg Platinol(r) (Bristol-Myers Squibb, New York, NY) in 1ml water and 2 ml purified medical grade sesame oil.

Intralesional 5-fluorouracil (1%) can also be administered in four or more sessions at two-week intervals.

Immunomodulation of Sarcoids using BCG

Topical tazarone gel (Tazorac, 0.1%; Allergan, Inc, Irvine, CA) (BID for seven days) followed by 5-fluorouracil (Efudix, 5%; Roche, Nutley, NJ) cream (BID for seven days) can shrink sarcoids in size and make the BCG therapy more efficacious. (Personal communication: Derek Knottenbelt, University of Liverpool, Liverpool, UK)

The sarcoid should be ultrasounded prior to BCG injection to identify the location of cystic abscesses. The injection of BCG into a cyst is ineffective at treating the sarcoid.

Using a 25-gauge hypodermic needle, 1 ml of BCG/cm^3 of tumor surface area is injected into the sarcoid lesion. Injection into sarcoid tissue is difficult, while cyst injection occurs with little resistance. Therapy is repeated at increasing one week intervals for up to 6 injections. Anaphylaxis may occur after the initial injection and can be minimized with pretreatment administration of flunixin meglumine (1.1 mg/kg IV) and systemically administered corticosteroids or diphenhydramine (0.05 to 1 mg/kg IV).

Interferon has been used for very aggressive equine sarcoids. Six to eight million IU given intravenously every three days for three weeks (7 injections total) is recommended.

II. SCC Therapy

Chemotherapy of invasive eyelid SCC with intralesional, slow release cisplatin has also been used with very effective results, with and without surgical debulking. One year relapse-free rates approach 90%. At least four sessions (and sometimes several more until tumor-free biopsy results are obtained) at 1-2 week intervals using 1 mg/cm3 of tumor is necessary. Tumors up to 20 cm^3 may be treated using 3.3 mg/ml cisplatin (10mg Platinol®) (Bristol-Myers Squibb, New York, NY) in 1 ml water and 2 ml purified medical grade sesame oil). If this therapeutic modality is chosen, the owner's must be committed to the entire course of therapy because if the injections are prematurely discontinued, the tumor that recurs often will be resistant to treatment thereafter.

Piroxicam (150 mg PO SID) can be beneficial in some ocular SCC. The drug is begun once a day and then reduced to every other day. Therapy with piroxicam should be continued for at least several months.

Topical 5-fluorouracil (1% 5-FU TID), or topical mitomycin C (0.02% QID) may be effective for corneal SCC in situ, and may be beneficial for extensive periocular SCC.

III. Ulcer Therapy

A. Antibiotics and Ulcers

Topically applied antibiotics, such as chloramphenicol, bacitracin-neomycin-polymyxin B, gentamicin, ciprofloxacin, or tobramycin ophthalmic solutions may be utilized initially to treat bacterial ulcers. Frequency of medication varies from q2h to q8h.

Cefazolin (55mg/ml), chloramphenicol, bacitracin, and carbenicillin are effective against beta hemolytic Streptococcus.

Ciprofloxacin, amikacin (10 mg/ml), and polymyxin B (0.25% IV solution) may be used topically for gentamicin resistant *Pseudomonas*.

B. Collagenolysis prevention with Ulcers

Serum can be administered topically as often as possible (q1h). Replace the serum every five days.

Five to 10 per cent acetylcysteine or 0.17% sodium EDTA can be instilled hourly, or by continuous lavage. Acetylcysteine breaks down the tear film layer and I no longer utilize it. Adding 10 ml of sterile water to a 10 ml purple topped vacutainer blood tube gives 0.17% EDTA.

It may be necessary to use serum, EDTA, and acetylcysteine simultaneously in severe cases.

Topical 0.1% doxycycline has anticollagenolytic benefits separate from its antimicrobial activity. It blocks TNF-alpha converting enzyme which is important in the activity of proteinases. Systemic doxycycline (10 mg/kg PO SID) may also be beneficial in treating melting ulcers.

The immune globulins found in tetanus antitoxin can be used subconjunctivally to reduce collagen breakdown.

C. Treating the Uveitis caused by an Ulcer

Atropine may be utilized topically q4h to q6h with the frequency of administration reduced as soon as the pupil dilates. Phenylephrine (2.5%) may be added to the topical atropine to dilate difficult pupils.

Horses receiving topically administered atropine should be monitored for signs of colic.

Topical nonsteroidal antiinflammatory drugs (NSAIDs) such as profenol, flurbiprofen and diclofenamic acid (BID to TID) can also reduce the degree of uveitis.

Topical corticosteroids are contraindicated for the treatment of uveitis caused by an ulcer. The use of systemic corticosteroids is debated but generally has little benefit and seems to cause no harm.

Systemically administered NSAIDs such as phenylbutazone (4.4 - 8.8mg/kg BID PO) or flunixin meglumine (1mg/kg BID, IV, IM or PO) can be used orally or parenterally. Flunixin appears more specific for eye pain in the horse.

Ranitidine (6.6 mg/kg PO TID) and sucralfate (20 mg/kg PO TID-QID), or omeprazole (4 mg/kg QD PO) may be needed for gastric ulcer prophylaxis when using systemic NSAID in foals.

D. Treatment Examples

Superficial Ulcers with Minimal Corneal Tissue Loss

Topical bacitracin-neomycin-polymyxin B or chloramphenicol QID

Topical Serum TID Atropine 1% BID or TID till pupil is dilated

Systemic NSAIDS (phenylbutazone or flunixin meglumine)

Recheck the next day to evaluate for "melting". Melting appears initially as a cloudiness at the ulcer margin.

Ulcers with Evidence of "Melting" or Keratomalacia (culture and cytology are highly recommended)

Topical tobramycin or gentamicin or ciprofloxacin or cefazolin q2h

Topical natamycin if cytology is positive for hyphae q4h

Topical atropine 3 to 4 times per day till pupil is dilated

Topical serum and/or other antiproteinases q1h

Systemic NSAIDS BID

Deep Ulcers, Descemetoceles and Perforated Ulcers

Continue aggressive medical therapy against infection and uveitis.

Consider culturing and use of fortified antibiotics (gentamicin 8mg/ml) or a change in antibiotics.

Conjunctival flap surgery is indicated as these types of ulcers need the fibroblasts, vascularization and physical support of a conjunctival flap to augment lost corneal thickness and increase strength.

Third eyelid flaps can be used to provide physical support of the weakened cornea.

Full thickness corneal perforations/lacerations with iris prolapse

Requires immediate suturing of the corneal lesion under general anesthesia.

Waiting to minimize "infection" is a mistake.

Medical therapy is still intensive both topically and systemically.

Enucleation may be indicated for corneal lesions > 15 mm in length, lacerations older than 2 weeks, and iris prolapses due to melting ulcers.

IV. Fungal Disease Therapy

A. Several options are available for treatment of fungal ulcers, fungal stromal abscesses, and fungal iris prolapses. Persistent ulcers should be cultured and corneal cytologic specimens examined.

Natamycin, 1% miconazole, 1% itraconazole/ 30% DMSO, 0.2% fluconazole, 0.15% amphotericin B (AMB), 2% povidone iodine solution, 0.2% chlorhexidine gluconate, posaconazole, voriconazole, and silver sulfadiazine can be utilized topically. Start therapy four to six times per day. Increase frequency of administration if necessary. Uveitis may be worse the day following initiation of antifungal therapy due to fungal death.

Systemically administered itraconazole (3 mg/kg BID PO) and fluconazole (1 mg/kg BID PO for 1 to 2 weeks, then QD for 1 to 2 weeks) can be useful in recalcitrant cases. Itraconazole does not appear to reach therapeutic levels in all cases.

B. Treatment Examples

Superficial fungal ulcer

Topical natamycin and miconazole QID

Topical 2% povidone iodine solution once per day (QD)

Topical bacitracin-neomycin-polymyxin B or chloramphenicol QID

Topical atropine 1% BID or TID till pupil is dilated

Topical Serum QID

Systemic NSAIDS (phenylbutazone or flunixin meglumine)

Recheck the next day to evaluate for "melting"

Fungal ulcer with stromal melting

Topical natamycin QID

Topical 2% povidone iodine solution QD

Topical gentamicin or tobramycin QID

Topical serum and/or other antiproteinases q1h

Atropine 1% BID or TID till pupil is dilated

Systemic NSAIDS (phenylbutazone or flunixin meglumine). Flunixin meglumine seems more able to reduce eye pain than other systemic NSAIDs, but also slows the healing corneal vascularization in many cases.

V. Stromal Abscess Therapy

A. Superficial Stromal Abscess Therapy

Medical therapy consists of aggressive use of topical and systemic antibiotics. Antifungal medications are also utilized topically for stromal abscesses.

Topical bacitracin-neomycin-polymyxin B or chloramphenicol QID

Topical natamycin or miconazole or voriconazole QID

Topical atropine 3 to 4 times per day initially

Systemic NSAIDs

Doxycycline 10 mg/kg PO BID or Trimethoprim sulfa 15-25 mg/kg PO BID

Surgery: Superficial scraping of epithelium QD

Consider intrastromal AMB (5 µg/0.1ml; multiple sites) in some stromal abscesses

B. Deep Stromal Abscess Therapy

Topical bacitracin-neomycin-polymyxin B or chloramphenicol QID

Topical natamycin and 1% miconazole QID

Topical atropine 3 to 4 times per day initially

Systemic flunixin meglumine (1mg/kg BID, IV, IM or PO)

Doxycycline 10 mg/kg PO BID or Trimethoprim sulfa 15-25 mg/kg PO BID

Systemically administered itraconazole (3 mg/kg BID PO) or fluconazole (1 mg/kg BID PO)

Corneal transplantation to remove the organisms or necrotic debris in the abscess can speed healing.

VI. ERU

A. Suppressing the Inflammation

Corticosteroids

Topical corticosteroids (1% prednisolone acetate or 0.1% dexamethasone) 4 to 6 times a day in early stages

Methylprednisolone acetate (40 mg every 1 to 3 weeks) and triamcinolone acetonide (40 mg every 1 to 3 weeks) can be utilized subconjunctivally in the horse.

Oral corticosteroids (prednisone 0.5 mg/kg q 24 h; dexamethasone 2-5 mg PO q 24 h) can be used in selected cases. Systemically administered dexamethasone (0.1 mg/kg PO, IM or IV SID) can be helpful.

Nonsteroidal Antiinflammatory Drugs

Flunixin meglumine (0.25 to 1.0 mg/kg BID, PO), phenylbutazone (1 gm BID, IV or PO), or aspirin (25 mg/kg BID, PO) are frequently used systemically to control intraocular inflammation. Methyl-sulfonylmethane (MSM; 0.06 mg/kg SID PO) is used in some cases in horses with ERU.

Ranitidine (6.6 mg/kg PO TID) and sucralfate (20 mg/kg PO TID-QID), or omeprazole (4 mg/kg QD PO) may be needed for gastric ulcer prophylaxis when using systemic NSAID in foals.

Flunixin meglumine seems more able to reduce eye pain than other systemic NSAIDs, but also slows corneal vascularization in some cases.

Topically administered NSAIDs such as diclofenac, flurbiprofen and suprofen may also be used to suppress signs of anterior uveitis.

Intravitreal or subconjunctival cyclosporine A sustained-release implants, or topical cyclosporine A may be beneficial.

B. Mydriasis/Cycloplegia

Topical atropine 2 to 3 times per day initially. 2.5% phenylephrine may need to be added topically to achieve mydriasis.

C. Antibiotics

Topical antibiotics (bacitracin-neomycin-polymyxin B or chloramphenicol) TID

Intravitreal gentamicin (4 mg/0.1ml) can benefit some ERU horses.

Antibiotic treatment for horses with positive titers for Leptospira remains speculative but streptomycin (11 mg/kg IM BID) may be a good choice for horses at acute and chronic stages of the disease. Penicillin G sodium (10,000 U/kg IV or IM QID) and tetracycline (6.6 - 11 mg/kg IV BID) at high dosages may be beneficial during acute leptospiral infections.

Tissue plasminogen activator (TPA) has been used to accelerate fibrinolysis and clear hypopyon and fibrin in the anterior chamber of horses with severe iridocyclitis. An intracameral injection of 50-150 micrograms/ eye can be made at the limbus with a 27-ga. needle under general anesthesia. TPA should be avoided if recent hemorrhage (<48h) is present.

D. Immunomodulation

Homeopathic remedies (eg, poultices of chamomile, and oral methylsulfonylmethane 15 mg/kg BID) for ERU have been used.

Acupuncture has been used to treat active ERU at the following acupoints once every three days:

ST1 (stomach meridian # 1): at the intersection between the medial and middle one third of the lower eyelid.

GB1 (gall bladder meridian # 1): 0.75cm lateral to the lateral canthus.

BL1 (bladder meridian # 1): at the medial canthus of the eye, in the indention dorsal to the base of the nictitating membrane.

Jing-shu (Eye association point): at the midpoint of the upper eyelid, ventral to the zygomatic process of the frontal bone.

Multivalent bovine leptospiral vaccines have been used in horses to treat intractable cases of ERU and to suppress herd outbreaks of leptospiral ERU, but their routine use as a preventative for ERU is controversial. The vaccinated horses remain serologically positive for leptospirosis.

VII. Glaucoma

A. Need to reduce IOP quickly

The topical miotics phospholine iodide (0.12-0.25% BID) and pilocarpine (2.0% QID), the beta-blocker timolol maleate (0.5 % BID), and the topical carbonic anhydrase inhbitor dorzo-lamine (2.0% TID) have been utilized singly or combined to lower IOP in horses with varying degrees of success. The newer prostaglandinoid glaucoma drugs should be avoided.

Isoxsuprine, a vasodilator used in navicular disease can be beneficial in selected equine glaucoma cases (0.6 mg/kg PO BID). The systemically administered carbonic anhydrase inhibitor acetazolamide (1-3 mg/kg QD, PO) can be used.

When medical therapy is inadequate, neodymium: yttrium-aluminum-garnet (Nd:YAG) laser cyclophotoablation may be a viable alternative for long-term IOP control and maintenance of vision. I recommend 55 laser sites per eye for contact Nd:YAG laser cyclophotoablation in the horse, 4-6 mm posterior to the limbus, at a power setting of 10 watts for 0.4 seconds duration per site. The anterior chamber may need to be tapped in some eyes post-laser.

Diode lasers may be used for contact transcleral cyclophotoablation. The diode laser is used at a power of 1500 mW and duration of 1500 msec per site. The treatments are done 4-6 mm posterior to the limbus in the dorsal, ventral and lateral quadrants. The nasal area is avoided. Complete circumferential lasering can damage the corneal sensory nerves resulting in a denervation keratopathy, corneal sloughing, and ulcer formation. I thus recommend only doing half the circumference per treatment (two treatments of 25 to 30 sites for a total treatment of 50-70 sites).

B. Treat Uveitis found with Glaucoma

Topically and systemically administered corticosteroids, and/or topically and systemically administered nonsteroidal antiinflammatories (phenylbutazone and flunixin meglumine), also appear to be beneficial in the control of IOP.

Use topical atropine with caution. It may cause sudden elevations in IOP.

Chronic glaucoma (blind eye)

Surgical therapy is usually required to prevent corneal ulceration caused by the inability of the lids to protect the cornea.

Enucleation/Intraocular prosthesis/ciliary body ablation with intravitreal gentamicin injection in blind painful eyes.

Ciliary body ablation: A frontal nerve block, sedation, a twitch, and topical 2.5% phenylephrine and proparacaine aid this procedure. I use a 20 gauge needle attached to a 3 cc syringe. The needle is inserted at a 45 degree angle 7 mm posterior to the dorsal limbus (left eye 1-2 o'clock; right eye 10-11 o'clock). Aspirate 1 ml of vitreous if the eye is hard, and then inject 0.5 to 1 ml of intravenous gentamicin. A severe uveitis will develop and cause globe phthisis. **This procedure is for blind eyes only!!**

VIII. Notes on Atropine

Topical atropine minimizes synechiae formation by inducing mydriasis, and alleviates some of the pain of anterior uveitis by relieving spasm of ciliary body muscles (cycloplegia). It also narrows the capillary inter-endothelial cell junctions to reduce capillary plasma leakage.

Although topically administered atropine can dilate the pupil over 14 days in the normal equine eye, its mydriatic/cyloplegic effect may be only a few hours in duration in the inflamed eye.

The ease with which mydriasis can be achieved with intermittent use of atropine is an important indication as to the stimulus intensity of the corneal ulcer or ERU.

Failure to achieve mydriasis with atropine indicates the stimulus for the uveitis is still present and quite prominent, and/or indicates the presence of synechiation.

Gut motility should be strictly monitored by abdominal auscultation and observation of signs of abdominal pain when using topically administered atropine in adult horses and foals, as gut motility can be markedly reduced by atropine in some horses. Should gut motility decrease during treatment with topically administered atropine, one can either discontinue the drug or change to the shorter acting tropicamide.

IX. Diagnostic Equipment/Drugs

Tropicamide 1% for mydriasis

Topical local anesthetic, scalpel blade and slides for cytology

Culture swabs

Lidocaine for nerve blocks

Fluorescein dye

Rose Bengal dye (available at http://www.akorn.com)

Schirmer tear strips*

Curved tip (#412) multipurpose nasolacrimal flush syringe

Direct Ophthalmoscope with cobalt blue filter

Finhoff transilluminator with 14 D lens*

Handheld slitlamp*

Tonopen or JonoVet tonometer*

Nasolacrimal lavage kit*

*optional

X. Surgical Procedures for Treatment of Corneal Injuries

Principles of Corneal microsurgery

A. Iris Prolapse

a. The corneal endothelium is very sensitive to mechanical trauma. When manipulating or holding corneal tissue, only the stroma and epithelium should be held with the corneal forceps.

b. Edges of corneal wounds are generally not debrided.

c. If an iris prolapse is fresh, an attempt is made to replace the protruding iris. If the iris tissue is damaged or necrotic, the protruding iris is excised with electrocautery. Hemorrhage is a risk if the iris is transected.

d. Partial thickness sutures (1/2 to 3/4 depth) are used in the cornea; full thickness penetrating sutures are never used.

e. The cornea is sutured with a simple interrupted pattern (1 mm apart); 5-0 to 8-0 Vicryl suture is best.

f. After partial closure of the wound, blood and fibrin clots in the anterior chamber are carefully removed by lavage, or more commonly digested with tissue plasminogen activator (50-150 micrograms).

g. Wound closure is completed and the anterior chamber reformed with hyaluronic acid, lactated Ringer's solution (LRS), or an air bubble.

B. Removal of Corneal Foreign Bodies

Corneal foreign bodies are removed in order to limit pain, reduce the potential for infection, and prevent vascularization and scar formation.

Small foreign bodies are removed with irrigation or a needle-shaped instrument.

After removal of the foreign body, a broad-spectrum topical antibiotic and atropine are administered to limit infection and control pain due to secondary uveitis.

C. Superficial Keratectomy

Superficial keratectomy is excision of the corneal epithelium and anterior stroma. Dissection is performed under magnification with a #64 Beaver or #15 Bard-Parker blade, and a Martinez corneal dissector.

Postoperative topical antibiotics and atropine are used to reduce infection and uveitis respectively.

D. Keratoplasty

The PLK, DLEK and PLK methods of corneal transplantation require meticulous surgical technique and postoperative care for success. They do have a high rate of tectonic success for iris prolapse, deep ulcers, and stromal abscesses.

Practice tips for PLK, DLEK, PK

1. Heal superficial ulcers before PLK surgery is done.

2. Make superficial PLK flaps 1 mm wider than the donor tissue on each side of the lesion. Abscess incisions should be 1 mm diameter larger than lesion.

3. Put viscoelastic on the iris surface as soon as the diseased deep tissue is removed.

4. Do not pull on debris in the anterior chamber.

5. Let IOP come down slowly or hyphema may occur.

6. Foal corneas are thin and may be incorporated into the recipient site faster.

7. Fibrin and acute pain several days after surgery can indicate an anterior chamber leak in PLK, DLEK and PK.

8. Check IOP and do Seidel's test postoperatively on a frequent basis.

9. Use serum topically postoperatively to minimize tear proteinase activity to protect the sutures in all three procedures.

10. The donor graft becomes clear for several weeks!

11. Do not handle superficial flap edges during surgery as bacterial infection can appear later.

12. Partially frozen grafts are easier to cut and to suture.

E. Conjunctival Pedicle Flap

Conjunctiva (excluding Tenon's capsule) can be used to aid healing of infected, melting, and deep or slow-healing corneal lesions.

Function of conjunctival flaps (CF): 1. Give structural support to corneal lesions; 2. Provide blood vessels for the vascular phase of corneal stromal healing; 3. Are a source of fibroblasts and connective tissue; 4. May inhibit tear film proteases as plasma from the leaking vessels of the flap percolates directly onto the wound.

Betadine solution (2.0%) is used to sterilize the eyelids and Cornea prior to surgery.

A conjunctival pedicle flap is made by incising the conjunctiva (excluding Tenon's capsule) 1-mm posterior to and parallel to the limbus with tenotomy scissors (figure 5.42). The distance of the limbus to the corneal lesion determines the length of this incision. The flap is undermined posteriorly toward the fornix. A perpendicular incision is made at the distal end of the flap, and an incision parallel to the first incision and limbus is made as wide as is necessary to cover the corneal lesion. The flap is rotated over the corneal defect and sutured in place with absorbable 5-0 to 7-0 suture in a simple interrupted pattern.

Practice tips for Conjunctival Flaps

1. Remove as much necrotic cornea as possible before placing graft. Make the flap thin.

2. Conjunctival flap (CF) fibrosis and failure may be associated with iris prolapse under the flap. Aqueous humor leakage induces fibroplasia of the corneal side of the flap such that this surface becomes thickened and fibrotic and does not completely adhere to the wound. The flap may still partially adhere but vascularization of the cornea may fail.

3. Flap bruising manifesting as purple areas of the CF may indicate ischemia conjunctival vessel necrosis.

4. A white flap has become avascular!

5. Flap bulging may indicate iris prolapse. Check for low IOP and perform a Seidel's test.

6. Continue anti-proteinases after flap placement or absorbable sutures may be dissolved prematurely.

8. Anchor flap with sutures at the limbus to reduce tension.

9. Streptococcus and Aspergillus can infect and melt a conjunctival flap!!

10. Flap color change from pink to purple, increased blepharospasm, and increased hypopyon indicate flap failure from aqueous humor toxicity. Perform a Seidel's test for a corneal micro leak.

F. Treatment of Descemetoceles

Descemetocele is the exposure of Descemet's membrane through a near full thickness defect in the corneal epithelium and stroma. The membrane may or may not protrude through the defect.

Due to the risk of rupture, a descemetocele is surgically repaired as soon as possible.

Careful debridement of infected or severely damaged ulcer margins speeds healing. Insertion of a donor corneal button into the defect adds support. The lesion will eventually vascularize and scar.

Use a conjunctival flap to both support the lesion and aid in vascularization.

Further support can be given with a temporary tarsorrhaphy or on occasion with a nictitans flap. Therapy with topical antibiotics and atropine, and systemic antibiotics and NSAIDs is used postoperatively.

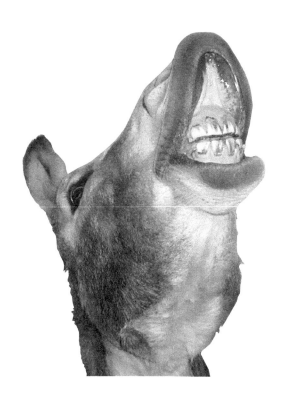

Index

Page numbers followed by an "f" indicate a figure.

Recommended Readings

Barnett KC, Crispin SM, Lavach JD, Matthews AG: Equine Ophthalmology: An Atlas and Text (2nd ed). Saunders, Edinburgh, 2004.

Berlin R, Eversbusch O: Zeitschrift für Vergleichende Augenheilkunde (Journal of Comparative Ophthalmology). FCW Vogel, Leipzig, pp 1-156, 1882.

Berlin R, Eversbusch O: Zeitschrift für Vergleichende Augenheilkunde II (Journal of Comparative Ophthalmology). FCW Vogel, Leipzig, pp 1-160, 1883.

Berlin R, Eversbusch O: Zeitschrift für Vergleichende Augenheilkunde III (Journal of Comparative Ophthalmology). FCW Vogel, Leipzig, pp 1-146, 1885.

Brooks DE, Matthews AG: Equine Ophthalmology, In Gelatt KN (ed), Veterinary Ophthalmology ed 4, Lippincott Williams and Wilkins, 2007.

Brooks DE: Guest Editor. Current Techniques in Equine Practice 4(1), 2005. Articles on ulcerative keratitis, cataract surgery, corneal transplantation, ERU, SCC, and ocular ultrasonography.

Carroll J, Murphy CJ, Neitz M, Ver Hoeve JN, Neitz J: Photopigment basis of dichromatic color vision in the horse. J of Vision 1(2): 80-87, 2001.

Dwyer AE, Crockett RS, Kalsow CM: Association of leptospiral seroreactivity and breed with uveitis and blindness in horses: 372 cases (1986-1993). Journal American Veterinary Medical Association 207(10): 1327-1331, 1995.

Equine Ophthalmology Supplement 2, Equine Veterinary Journal, November, 1983.

Equine Ophthalmology Supplement 10, Equine Veterinary Journal, September, 1990.

Fruhauf B, Ohnesorge B, Deegen E, Boeve M: Surgical management of equine recurrent uveitis with single port pars plana vitrectomy. Veterinary Ophthalmology 1(2-3): 137-152, 1998.